Qualitative Methods for Health Research

INTRODUCING QUALITATIVE METHODS provides a series of volumes which introduce qualitative research to the student and beginning researcher. The approach is interdisciplinary and international. A distinctive feature of these volumes is the helpful student exercises.

One stream of the series provides texts on the key methodologies used in qualitative research. The other stream contains books on qualitative research for different disciplines or occupations. Both streams cover the basic literature in a clear and accessible style, but also cover the 'cutting edge' issues in the area.

SERIES EDITOR
David Silverman (Goldsmiths College)

EDITORIAL BOARD
Michael Bloor (University of Wales, Cardiff)
Barbara Czarniawska (University of Gothenburg)
Norman Denzin (University of Illinois, Champaign)
Barry Glassner (University of Southern California)
Jaber Gubrium (University of Missouri)
Anne Murcott (South Bank University)
Jonathan Potter (Loughborough University)

TITLES IN SERIES

Qualitative Methods for Health Research

Judith Green
and
Nicki Thorogood

SAGE Publications
London • Thousand Oaks • New Delhi

© Judith Green and Nicki Thorogood 2004

First published 2004

Apart from any fair dealing for the purposes of research or private study, or criticism or review, as permitted under the Copyright, Designs and Patents Act, 1988, this publication may be reproduced, stored or transmitted in any form, or by any means, only with the prior permission in writing of the publishers, or in the case of reprographic reproduction, in accordance with the terms of licences issued by the Copyright Licensing Agency. Inquiries concerning reproduction outside those terms should be sent to the publishers.

 SAGE Publications Ltd
1 Oliver's Yard
55 City Road
London EC1Y 1SP

SAGE Publications Inc.
2455 Teller Road
Thousand Oaks, California 91320

SAGE Publications India Pvt Ltd
B-42, Panchsheel Enclave
Post Box 4109
New Delhi 100 017

British Library Cataloguing in Publication data

A catalogue record for this book is available from the British Library

ISBN 0 7619 4770 1
ISBN 0 7619 4771 X (pbk)

Library of Congress number 2003115334
Typeset by Keyword Publishing Services Ltd, Wallington, Surrey
Printed in Great Britain by The Cromwell Press Ltd, Trowbridge, Wiltshire

Contents

Case Studies

Preface

There are a number of excellent introductory textbooks available on qualitative research, so the decision to produce yet another one perhaps needs justifying. We have written this one in response to frequent requests from our students, who are predominantly postgraduates with considerable professional experience but little prior knowledge of the social sciences. They come from almost all countries in the world, and want an introduction to qualitative methods that is sensitive to the practicalities of doing sound research on health topics in a wide variety of settings. Although the principles of research design and conduct may be the same wherever it is happening, and whatever the topic studied, clearly the practice is not. First, the context of health research may be rather different from that of general social research. It is increasingly undertaken within multi-disciplinary teams, in which the legitimacy of using qualitative methodologies is still challenged. It is undertaken in institutional contexts (medical schools, health authorities, hospitals) in which the assumed model of research may be clinical, rather than social. Although none of this has any impact on the principles of 'doing good research', it does demand a particular range of skills from the researcher, including the ability to explain those principles to a wide range of collaborators and potential users, and an understanding of why the most common conflicts over issues such as research design may occur. Second, most of the social research texts on the market assume a Western setting, and it may be difficult for a reader to grasp the principles if their initial reaction is 'But that wouldn't work in my country!' The first incentive for producing this text was, then, to provide an introduction to qualitative methods that used examples of health research from a number of different settings, so that we can demonstrate how key methodological issues may have different implications in different contexts. We have been aided in this task by colleagues from the London School of Hygiene and Tropical Medicine who work across the world, and we have used examples from their research liberally to illustrate key points.

Having taught methodology courses to students from a range of low-, middle- and high-income countries, we have realized that there is a huge amount to learn from reflecting on the differences and similarities between what is possible and productive in diverse contexts. Being forced to reflect on, for instance, different assumptions made about research interviews can aid an awareness of the cultural specificity of the interview format in any setting –

something we can easily forget if all our interviewees share similar cultural backgrounds to ourselves. Thinking through how the methodological aims may be shaped by practical constraints can be a very useful way of clarifying exactly what our aims are in using particular designs, or particular methods of collecting data. Confronting examples from work in different settings helps all of us challenge our assumptions about what we are trying to do in conducting qualitative research of and for health.

A second incentive for writing this book was to bridge a gap that is sometimes apparent between policy-orientated field guides that aim to provide 'toolboxes' for novice researchers and theoretical introductions to social research that may appear to have little relevance to researchers working in applied areas. A key argument of this book is that good-quality applied qualitative work *has* to be theoretically informed: doing policy-orientated studies is no excuse for poor design, or inadequate attention to methodology. But it is not always obvious how this is to be done, particularly if faced with the constraints of short-term funding or inadequate training in social science methods. We hope this book will help more practically minded researchers to see the value of attending to theoretical issues, both for producing more useful findings and for unpacking some of the debates they will inevitably have about the validity, generalizability and implications of their findings.

Following from this, a third aim of this book is to explore the contribution of qualitative methods to understanding health and health behaviour. Although there is now largely an acceptance of the value of qualitative methods in public health research, many of our students and colleagues still report having to 'justify' their use to collaborators who are sceptical or simply poorly informed. Qualitative researchers still face questions about the validity and generalizability of their methods, and lack of understanding of what qualitative research aims to do. Throughout this book we have suggested how this kind of scepticism can be met – not to convince our readers, who are presumably already convinced, but to help in potential discussions with colleagues from other research traditions.

This book is intended primarily, then, for public health, primary care, health promotion and nursing practitioners and managers, in both developed and developing countries, with little previous experience of social science theory, who need to commission, use or conduct qualitative research. The aims are to introduce readers to some of the debates in qualitative methodology, to demonstrate the uses of qualitative designs and methods of data generation in a wide range of health research projects, and to suggest ways of improving their own research practice. We also hope it will be a useful text for social research students, in introducing some of the particular methodological possibilities and challenges of researching health.

The structure of the book is straightforward. The chapters in Part 1 deal with methodological principles, research designs and ethics. They introduce some of the key terms used in methodology, and some of the underlying principles of qualitative approaches. Those in Part 2 discuss four common strategies for producing or collecting qualitative data: in-depth interviews, group interviews, observation and documentary research. These chapters provide overviews of these methods of generating data and suggestions for improving research practice. The final chapter in this section is an introduction to some common ways of analysing qualitative data. Part 3 highlights the practical issues raised by 'doing' qualitative health research, with chapters on working in multi-disciplinary settings and on writing and reading qualitative work. Throughout the book we have drawn on examples of social research on health from a number of settings. Some of these are extended case studies, which are summaries of published research. It would be helpful to look at the sources of these wherever possible, as a good way of learning about methods is to read how others have approached questions of design and conduct. Even better as a learning tool is *doing* research, and there are suggestions for exercises to develop your own skills at the end of each chapter.

Finally, we should like to acknowledge the input of our past and current colleagues and students from the London School of Hygiene and Tropical Medicine, whose experiences, both published and unpublished, have been drawn on widely in writing this book. We are particularly grateful to: the students who have taken Qualitative Methodologies over the last few years, whose lively discussions and comments have contributed to many of the ideas here (often in ways they may not approve of!); Helen Marshall, for comments on several chapters; Simon Lewin and Gillian Hundt, whose research experiences have been drawn on in a number of chapters; Geraldine Barrett, for her contributions to Chapter 8; and Simon Carter, for contributions to Chapter 10.

Judith Green and Nicki Thorogood

Part 1

Principles and Approaches in Qualitative Health Research

1

Qualitative Methodology and Health Research

CHAPTER SUMMARY

This chapter first introduces the theoretical perspectives that have generated qualitative research both into and for health, and argues that an understanding of these is vital for both conducting good-quality research and for researching in a multi-disciplinary environment. Some broad orientations common to much qualitative research are then outlined. The contribution of qualitative research to disciplines such as public health, health promotion and health services research is discussed.

Introduction: health research

'Health' and 'illness' have long been topics of interest for social science disciplines such as sociology, social anthropology and history.

- *Sociology* is the study of human society. It has traditionally focused on developed countries, with the sociology of health and illness addressing such issues as concepts of health and illness, inequalities in health, experiences of health and health care systems (Annandale 1998).

- *Social anthropology*, the study of people in the context of culture and society, has traditionally studied cultures 'other' than that of the researcher. Medical anthropologists have focused on how a society's beliefs and practices relating to health and illness (including healing systems and folk practices) are embedded in other aspects of its culture (Helman 1984).
- *History of medicine* has contributed to understanding the history of medicine and medical knowledge, understanding the role of health and illness in social history, and to policy studies in the health arena (James 1994).

Maintaining health and dealing with ill health are universal challenges, and there is now a large research literature within these disciplines on how these have been accomplished over time and across different human societies. Health professionals have a long history of integrating insights from social science research into their understanding of human health (see, for instance, Henderson 1935; Kleinman 1973; Helman 1984). More recently, the *methods* of social research have become an accepted part of health research in areas such as public health, primary care, health promotion and nursing. Disciplines such as sociology, social anthropology and history have their own methodological traditions, but have in common perhaps a focus on human behaviour in context, whether social, cultural or historical. Health care practitioners, managers and policy-makers have increasingly turned to the qualitative methods of social inquiry used within the social sciences to enhance understanding of health, health behaviour and health services, and to improve the management and provision of health services. As the problems of public health are increasingly those of human behaviour, rather than the development of new technical interventions, those trained primarily in health sciences, such as medicine or nursing, are turning to social research to help understand how to improve health and health care. This book is intended for both qualitative social scientists interested in applying their disciplines to health research, and for health professionals interested in using qualitative research approaches.

We focus on the particular contribution of qualitative research methods to health research. What we mean by 'health research' includes two broad strands of work. First are critical studies *of* health from various social science perspectives, which address questions such as: What are health and illness? How are they managed, and in whose interests? Second are studies *for* health, from within the disciplines of public health, health promotion or health services research, in which the contributions of social science are defined in terms of the health agenda. The distinction between these two sorts of investigation is perhaps a useful one for thinking about the aims of the study (is it basic research, aiming to expand our knowledge of society, or applied research, aiming to address an existing health care problem?). How the two kinds of investigation are written up may also differ, in order to meet the expectations of different intended audiences (see Chapter 10). However, the distinction does not imply different criteria for methodological rigour. Doing applied research *for* health is not an excuse for inadequate research design, a superficial approach to data collection or under-theorized analysis. Producing useful findings involves, as a necessary condition, producing sound findings. Indeed, if the research has been funded to produce policy-relevant findings, there is perhaps even more reason for rigorous design and analysis. The principles of qualitative research are, therefore, exactly the same, whether the study is primarily academic (such as a PhD thesis in Anthropology) or more 'applied', such as a funded evaluation of a health care project. Similarly, the same principles of good design and conduct apply whether the research setting is a health service organization in a high-income country, or a rural village in a low-income country. Clearly the practicalities of carrying out the study will differ, but we hope to show how the same elements of research planning are involved. Whatever the setting, the researcher has to consider the local cultural and social context, and this is an essential part of adapting methodological techniques to a particular research project. Throughout this book we have used examples from a variety of settings, and we hope this range will illustrate the universal applicability of methodological principles.

What is qualitative research?

Health research, then, includes any study addressing understandings of human health, health behaviour or health services, whatever the disciplinary starting point. What is meant by 'qualitative' research is perhaps more contentious. Some have seen the division between 'quantitative' and 'qualitative' approaches as a false one, and it is perhaps impossible (and unhelpful) to characterize qualitative research in a way that is completely separate from quantitative research. Although qualitative research tends to use language data (written or oral), and quantitative research numerical data, for instance, this is not always the case. Many qualitative studies use simple frequency counts, whereas language data can be used in quantitative studies. Although qualitative research tends to have smaller sample sizes, it certainly does not follow that any study with a small sample is a qualitative study.

There are some methods of data collection that are particularly associated with qualitative methods. These are discussed in the chapters in Part 2 of this book. However, these methods of data collection can also be used in quantitative studies, so it is not merely the way in which data are collected (such as through an interview, or by observation) that characterizes a study as qualitative. It might be more useful to characterize qualitative research not by the kind of data produced or the methods used to produce them, but by the overall aims of the study. The most basic way of characterizing qualitative studies is that those aims are generally to seek answers to questions about the 'what', 'how' or 'why' of a phenomenon, rather than questions about 'how many' or 'how much'. Box 1.1 shows some examples of qualitative research studies reported in social science and biomedical journals, together with their main methods of data collection and the stated aims of the study.

Box 1.1   Some examples of qualitative health research questions

Title of paper	Methods of data collection	Aims
Guinea worm: an in-depth study of what happens to mothers, families and communities (Watts et al. 1989)	In-depth interviews, observations	'exploring the processes associated with incapacity due to guinea worm and its impact on the community'
Cancer patients' information needs and help-seeking behaviour (Leydon et al. 2000)	In-depth interviews	'to explore why cancer patients do not want or seek information about their condition other than that supplied by physicians'
Doctor in the house (Hardey 1999)	Household interviews	'[to examine] the internet as a source of knowledge about health in relation to the broader sociological debates about deprofessionalization and consumerism'
Leprosy among the Limba (Opala and Boillot 1996)	In-depth interviews	'examines Limba concepts of leprosy within the wider context of Limba world view'
Parents' perspectives on the MMR immunisation (Evans et al. 2001)	Focus group interviews	'to investigate what influences parents' decisions on whether to accept or refuse . . . [measles, mumps and rubella] immunisation'

Note that many of the studies in Box 1.1 have 'explore' as an aim, suggesting a need to understand more about a phenomenon, rather than 'measure' it. These studies aim to investigate health, illness or health services from the perspective of the communities and individuals affected, or the professionals who provide health services for them. Understanding questions such as these as legitimate aims for research is the consequence of having a particular theoretical perspective on the role of knowledge, how we acquire it from research activities, and what 'counts' as valid knowledge about the world. Although theoretical assumptions in research articles are not often made explicit, they nonetheless frame the kinds of questions researchers decide to ask, how they go about answering them, and how debates about the soundness of their findings are conducted. Therefore, a consideration of the theoretical approaches and broad orientations that are typical of qualitative approaches is fundamental to understanding the contribution of qualitative research to the study of health.

Theoretical approaches

'Theory' is central to research, even the most applied research, at a number of levels. First, there are what could be called large-scale, or macro, theories about the social world and how it works.

Macro and middle-range theories

'Macro' theoretical perspectives frame particular issues as 'puzzles' or questions requiring research because they entail particular assumptions about the way the world is, and how people behave within it. These might include questions such as: Is it inevitable that wealth is unequally distributed? Is there a real world of physical objects that exist separately from and independently of our perceptions of them? One well-known example of macro-theory is the *materialist approach*, which is built on an assumption that the material sphere of life (such as economic relations) determines other aspects, such as culture. In this tradition, Karl Marx developed his theory of class relations to explain both the contemporary situation and to predict future social patterns. The basis of his theory was the inevitable conflict produced between those who *own* the means of generating wealth (the means of production) – that is, the ruling class – and those who have to sell their labour – that is, the working class. This is an economic theory of production using generalizable concepts.

It is, nevertheless, not the only way of explaining that particular set of social relations, and other economists, Adam Smith for example, observed the same phenomena (the effects of industrialization) and theorized that the division was not only inevitable, but also that it was uncontentious. Other social theorists (rather than economists) working at a similar period to Marx also produced explanations of these conditions but proposed that the social processes to which they gave rise were a matter of consensus between the different interest groups. Thus one of the major divisions in social theory has been between those who take a 'conflict' and those who take a 'consensus' perspective. Clearly this initial position about the way in which the social world works will lead to very different ideas about how to make sense of other social phenomena, and indeed whether they are even framed as puzzles or problems at all. Thus, if you take a Marxist view of industrial relations, conflict between workers and bosses, for example in the form of strikes, would seem entirely expected – and harmonious periods of production would be puzzling and might suggest a modification of the theory was needed. In contrast, a consensus theorist would feel that a period of dispute was an anomaly. Large-scale, or macro, theory allows questions to be asked at the higher level of social organization. Examples would include questions about the relationship between social class and ill health, or indeed poverty and ill health, or about the effects of globalization, or if 'globalization' is a phenomenon that exists.

A larger set of presumptions or particular world-view will, then, frame any social inquiry. For the most part, however, these remain implicit. Few researchers state the assumptions they have about the social order, and why these have shaped their particular research question as a legitimate one, or as a puzzle that needs explaining. Nevertheless, we believe it is important to bear in mind that all researchers will have a particular world-view, or theoretical perspective, which both underpins and shapes their project and its findings.

As well as shaping inquiry at the most abstract level, macro-theory also generates what we could call 'middle-range theories' that link concepts together, and sometimes generate hypotheses to be tested, or interesting questions to address. Middle-range theories are the link between the general, abstract concepts of macro-theory (social class, gender, globalization and so on) and the grounded, observable behaviour of people in everyday settings. Thus, in understanding specific social issues, such as ill health, the concepts of 'health' or 'illness' that are employed will generally be derived from a larger-scale, if taken for granted, theory about the way the world works. These might lead to questions such as: What is the relationship between employment and health? Or, are women's experiences of health care different from those of men? In Box 1.1, for instance, the aims of Hardey's (1999) study of how people use the Internet to access health information explicitly cite debates about 'deprofessionalization and consumerism'. These are middle-range theoretical concepts he has drawn on to generate research questions. How users of the Internet use the information they find becomes an interesting question in the light of theories about deprofessionalization (that, for instance, the power of medicine is in decline because of the public's greater access to health knowledge) and consumerism (that treating health as any other commodity may change the ways in which we access health care). Often, researchers are not explicit about the theoretical underpinnings of their research, although theoretical concerns are implicit in the aims. Take another study listed in Box 1.1, Leydon et al.'s (2000) study of the information needs of cancer patients, for instance. Here, the research question derives in part from an assumption in Western health care that patients want, and ought, to know as much as they can about their own illnesses. There is a body of middle-range theory that addresses communication in health care settings and the needs of patients for information, and this generates a set of possible research questions around patients' needs for information and how these needs are met.

Middle-range theories are often rooted in particular disciplines, and we acquire our knowledge of them through training as nurses, doctors, sociologists, psychologists and so on. For example, if we take the study listed in Box 1.1 by Maggie Evans and colleagues on how parents make a decision to have their children immunized, there are a number of theoretical approaches that might have had relevance. Each would imply a rather different research question, and different ways of finding out the answer. Box 1.2 suggests, in summary form, some 'middle-range theories' associated with particular disciplines or professional knowledge that might influence other studies on this topic.

The suggested questions are all potentially interesting and legitimate, but our professional and academic training means that we are more familiar with some of these bodies of theory than others. When we are considering a particular topic, we draw upon these explanations (of how professionals and clients relate, or how individuals make decisions) to shape specific questions that are interesting because they relate to a broader body of theory. Social science disciplines such as sociology and psychology tend to be more explicit about these kinds of theory than biomedical sciences, but health professionals also have a set of more or less formal explanatory models they draw on to make sense of topics as research questions. The advantages and challenges of working across disciplines, when we are often combining not just methods of data collection, but also these kinds of theoretical approaches, are discussed in Chapter 9.

As an example of how middle-range theory informs both the framing of particular issues as research problems, and the ways in which we can understand them, consider the example of Rachel Jewkes and colleagues' (1998) work on

---

Box 1.2   Researching parents' decisions about childhood immunizations: possible theoretical starting points for research

Middle-range theory	Possible research questions	Main discipline
The *health belief model* (Becker 1974) suggests that the likelihood of an individual engaging in a particular behaviour results from their assessment of the costs and benefits of that action, and their perceived vulnerability to illness	What risks and benefits do parents associate with the immunization? How susceptible do they think children are to measles, mumps and rubella?	Psychology
Lack of 'compliance' with health advice reflects, in part, failures of health professional–client communication	Are parents more likely to 'comply' with immunizations if they have an opportunity to discuss their worries with a health professional?	General practice
There is a 'lay epidemiology' (Rogers and Pilgrim 1995) of risks associated with immunizations that may be different from that of experts	What sources of knowledge do parents draw on to assess the risks of immunization? How do experts and non-professionals explain risks?	Sociology

nurse–patient interactions in South African obstetric public health services. Jewkes et al. found evidence of widespread abuse of patients by nurses, including clinical neglect, scolding, humiliating, and even slapping women in labour. Although widely recognized as a 'problem' in South Africa, and commonly talked about by both patients and nurses they interviewed, it had not been recognized as a policy problem by professional organizations, nor had it been the object of research aimed at finding solutions. That the researchers could frame what is presumably an everyday feature of normal life as a research question ('Why do nurses abuse patients?') relies first of all on a body of nursing theory that constructs the nurse's role as one of caring, nurturing and compassion. Without a normative theory of how things 'should' be (that is, nurses should be caring, not abusive), the behaviour they documented could not be constructed as a problem to be understood. Second, although participants' accounts focused on personal characteristics of individual nurses as the cause of the problem, the researchers could draw on a number of theoretical perspectives to make sense of the problem in a way that suggested particular solutions. These included accounts of the ethnic and class basis of South African social structure, which makes the nurses' social position precarious; in this kind of social context, abusing patients may be one route for symbolically stressing the social distance between themselves and their patients.

Theories of knowledge

A third level of theory that researchers have to consider relates to theories of knowledge, or ideas about how we come to *know* the world, and have faith in the truth, or validity, of that knowledge. The theory of knowledge belongs to a branch of philosophy called *epistemology*. As research is essentially about producing knowledge about the world that we can claim as valid, some attention to epistemology is vital. Different epistemological traditions imply different ways of 'knowing' the world, and rather different accounts of the status of that knowledge. Most societies, for instance, include healers from a number of traditions who base their work on very different epistemologies; that is, different understandings of what leads to health or illness, different understandings of how the body works, and different understandings of how the healer can diagnose a problem. An illustration comes from a series called 'Second Opinion', that ran in the *Observer* newspaper, which used this contrast in a weekly article from two practitioners, one a general practitioner with a bio-medical training, the other an Ayurvedic practitioner. Box 1.3 illustrates how the different epistemological assumptions of the two approaches lead to very different advice for potential clients.

There are clear implications for health research in these contrasting understandings of 'health' and what it is. If, for example, these two practitioners wanted to research the efficacy of their remedies, they would be asking slightly different questions. The biomedically trained GP may be more interested in how the drugs reduce symptoms framed by a biomedical understanding of the

---

Box 1.3   How to deal with rheumatoid arthritis: different epistemological approaches

	Biomedically trained general practitioner	Ayurvedic practitioner
Cause	'the body produces antibodies to its own immunoglobulins'	'aggravated vata (air element) combined with an increase in ama or toxins in the body'
Advice	'rehabilitation programme of exercise, physiotherapy and patient education designed to improve muscle strength, encourage mobility and prevent depression'	'Panchakarma, a detoxification and rejuvenation treatment . . . oil massage with mahanaraya oil . . . a vata balancing diet with rice, vegetables and lentils'
Prognosis	'. . . there is no cure . . . and a high incidence of serious side effects from drugs'	'good results . . . [from] an anti-arthritic formula [of] anti-inflammatory herbs'

Source: *Observer Magazine*, 30 June 2002.

'disease' of arthritis, whereas the Ayurvedic practitioner might be interested in how well remedies detoxify the body. Understanding how different disciplinary traditions generate different legitimate research questions and different ways of convincingly answering them is key to working in multi–disciplinary settings. However, it is not always as easy to identify the different frameworks used by researchers as it is to identify the kinds of differences outlined in the box between different healing traditions, because they are rarely explicitly discussed, or set out as an obvious contrast. *Many debates about the value of research findings are rooted in epistemological differences between researchers in terms of what kind of knowledge they believe research should produce, or what counts as adequate evidence for conclusions to be drawn.* For this reason, it is worth outlining some of the main epistemological starting points of research, to help unpack the assumptions on which research knowledge is built. These will help understand the kinds of knowledge produced by qualitative research, and the particular contribution they make. Many of the epistemological assumptions of qualitative research arise from a critique of 'positivism'; that is, an approach to knowledge rooted in what early social scientists saw as the methods of the natural sciences.

Positivism

Over the last few hundred years the natural sciences, and many of the more quantitative social sciences, have developed a broad view of science and knowledge that has been described as 'positivism'. A positivist philosophy is one that assumes that there is a stable reality 'out there' – that phenomena (such as diseases, bacteria, villages, health) exist whether we are looking at them or not, and that they exist in exactly the same way whether we understand them or not. Thus, human understanding may be flawed (in, for instance, believing malaria to be caused by 'bad air'), but there is a potential 'right' explanation that we are getting closer to as understanding of health and disease increases. The implications of this starting point for research methods are threefold. First, there is a stress on *empiricism*, or studying only observable phenomena. At the beginning of the 'scientific revolution', this was an innovation, in terms of replacing the philosophical speculations of pre-Enlightenment scientists with a science grounded in the experimental method and on observations of the natural world. The second implication is known as the *unity of method*, the idea that eventually, when mature, all sciences will share the same methods of inquiry. At this point of maturity, the proper object of scientific inquiry is the establishment of relationships of cause and effect and the generation of laws about the natural world. That many of the social sciences focus on other questions is, in this view, evidence of their immaturity. Because we understand, as yet, little about human behaviour, we have not got to the point where we can look for relationships between cause and effect. A third element of a positivist approach is the emphasis on *value-free inquiry*. Science is held to be separate from society, and as objective, rational and neutral. In this view, knowledge derived from proper scientific inquiry is not bound up with emotional, subjective or political viewpoints, and is 'true' for all times and places.

This model of scientific inquiry has come under considerable criticism, from both those who see it as an idealized model of how scientific progress happens and those who see it as an inappropriate model for research, particularly social research. In the qualitative social sciences, research is often rooted in rather different epistemological traditions, which depart from one or more tenets of positivism.

Interpretative approaches

Some have seen a positivist view as an unachievable and inappropriate goal for research into human behaviour. Human beings differ in some essential respects from the objects of natural science inquiry. Unlike atoms (or plants or planets), human beings make sense of their place in the world, have views on researchers who are studying them, and behave in ways that are not determined in law-like ways. They are complex, unpredictable, and reflect on their behaviour. Therefore, the methods and aims of the natural sciences are unlikely to be useful for studying people and social behaviour: instead of explaining people and society, research should aim to understand human behaviour. This is the starting point of the *interpretative approach*. In this view, the most interesting questions are not about the 'reality' of the world, but about people's interpretations of it. Thus, if we were interested in how people took medication for their asthma, we might be more interested not in any objective reality of severity of symptoms, but rather in patients' interpretations of their symptoms, since these may tell us more about how they use medication. This interpretative tradition characterizes much qualitative work in health research, which focuses on the meaning of phenomena (such as symptoms, health behaviours) for people. Case Study 1.1 illustrates an example of research in this tradition. The aim of interpretative research is an understanding of the world from the point of view of participants in it, rather than an explanation of the world.

Many other case studies throughout this book draw on interpretative approaches. Case Study 5.2, for instance, summarizes a study of how people interpret media messages about HIV and AIDS. Case Study 8.1 describes research on the meaning of glaucoma diagnoses and symptoms for patients.

Social constructionism

A second criticism of positivist assumptions that has informed much qualitative work is a more philosophical one that questions the view that there is one stable, pre-existing reality 'out there' waiting to be discovered. Instead, reality is held to be socially constructed. How we divide up the world (for instance, how we see the systems of the body, or how we classify diseases) is the result of historical, social and political processes, rather than an inevitable result of our greater understanding of the 'reality' of the body, or disease. This leads to a second qualitative tradition: the *social constructionist* (sometimes called 'constructivist') approach. The proper object of research from this perspective is thus how phenomena are constructed: what are the processes by which diseases become classified in particular ways, who has the power to produce legitimate classifications, and what are the implications of such classifications? There is a strong tradition of constructionism in the qualitative social sciences in health, which has had a vital role in questioning common-sense assumptions about the categories we use routinely, as if they were 'natural' categories, rather than social ones. One example is described in Case Study 7.1, which shows how Sudden Infant Death Syndrome can be analysed as a socially constructed category.

The constructionist approach, although an influential one in qualitative research, has not been without its critics. Mike Bury (1986), for instance, takes issue with the relativism implied by an extreme constructionist position, claiming it poses a logical difficulty. If phenomena such as disease categories are merely 'social constructions', he argues, rather than categories of the natural world, how are we to derive knowledge of them, other than through similarly constituted social categories? There is no rational basis to make a claim for producing valid knowledge of socially constructed phenomena, as there is no sense in which the researcher can 'stand outside' the constructions that he or she is analysing. Bury warns that an extreme agnosticism about the natural world can mean that 'reality is portrayed as a contingent and haphazard affair' (Bury 1986:155). In the arena of health and illness, where research deals with

Case Study 1.1   Using qualitative research to explore patient understandings of asthma

(Source: Adams, S., Pill, R. and Jones, A. (1997) 'Medication, chronic illness and identity: the perspectives of people with asthma', *Social Science and Medicine*, 45: 189–201)

Asthma is a common condition, and from the perspective of health professionals, there is a problem in that many patients don't take medication as prescribed: the medication intended to prevent symptoms (the 'preventor') may not be taken at all, and the medication intended to relieve symptoms (the 'reliever') is often over-used. The authors of this paper note that such apparently irrational behaviour is understandable if we look at the patients' perspective – how they understand symptoms and medications, and how they are managed within everyday lives. The study used in-depth interviews with a sample of patients on preventative asthma medication. After analysing patients' accounts, the researchers identified three broad groups in their sample.

First were the 'deniers'. These patients, about half of the sample, denied that they had asthma, although they had been identified from general practice records as people diagnosed with asthma and prescribed preventative medication. However, these patients did not see themselves as asthmatic, but saw their problems as 'chest trouble' or bronchitis. They also claimed that symptoms did not interfere with everyday life, despite at times using quite complex or drastic strategies to manage symptoms, such as complete avoidance of going outdoors. This group also hid their medication use to a large extent, reporting only using inhalers out of sight of others, and had negative views of asthmatics – an identity they did not accept for themselves. Most did not use preventative medications at all – partly because of worry that they would become dependent on drugs that have to be taken daily, but also because taking medication regularly, whether there are symptoms or not, relies on accepting an asthmatic identity, which these 'deniers' did not. Given that they didn't see themselves as having asthma, they did not attend special clinics for asthma.

A smaller group within the sample accepted both the diagnosis and their doctors' advice completely, using medications as prescribed and taking pride in doing so. For this group, the route to 'normal life' was gaining adequate control over symptoms through medication. Their definitions of asthma coincided with those of medical professionals. For them, 'asthmatic' was not a stigmatized identity, and they used inhalers in public.

The final group was identified as the 'pragmatists'. This group did use preventative medication, usually not as prescribed, however, but only when their asthma was particularly bad. They also had a pragmatic approach to disclosing asthma diagnosis; for instance, in telling family but not employers in case it prejudiced their employment prospects. This group accepted they had asthma, but usually perceived it as mild, or as an acute rather than chronic illness.

Looking at medication use from the point of view of patients enabled the researchers to see how health behaviour was tied tightly to people's beliefs about asthma and what kind of chest problems they had, as well as social circumstances and the threat of an asthmatic identity to other social identities. For service providers and health promoters, this kind of information is very useful. First it suggests that providing designated asthma clinics may not appeal to the majority of sufferers, since they don't identify themselves as having asthma. Second, professionals can see that what appears to be irrational use of medication, and the result of ignorance, is actually deeply embedded in complex social identities that have to be managed. For patients, health, defined in medical terms, may not be the top priority all the time, and the meaning of symptoms for professionals may be rather different from the meaning of symptoms for patients.

phenomena such as distress, pain and death, such an extreme view, he suggests, is untenable and unhelpful.

How far along the 'constructionist' approach an individual researcher stands is, perhaps, largely a matter of their *a priori* assumptions about the nature of reality. It is impossible to 'test' the extent to which phenomena exist independently of our attempts to study them. A social constructionist approach does, though, generate rather different possible questions about a research topic. To follow on from the example of asthma in Case Study 1.1, for instance, rather than asking 'How do people cope with asthma?' or 'How do patients interpret symptoms?', a social constructionist research study might start with questions such as 'How and why did "asthma" emerge as a category of disease?' (see Gabbay 1982 for one perspective on this) or 'How do some people come to be defined as "asthma patients"?' Even if questions like these are not core to the research, they can be very useful for sensitizing researchers to be critical of the categories they do use.

Interpretative approaches, then, start with a different aim from positivist ones — that of understanding, rather than explaining, reality. Constructionist approaches go further, in taking issue with the very concept of a pre-existing reality.

Critical approaches

A third set of criticisms of positivism have questioned the 'value-free' description of the scientific process on two levels:

1   First, because it is an *idealistic* view, in that 'scientific research' is in itself a social process, carried out by humans within specific social contexts, so it cannot be separate from or outside our social world (that is, research *can't* be value-free).
2   Second, because it is a morally indefensible position. There are some perspectives, for example some feminist and participatory approaches, that explicitly assume research should have a political goal as well as a purely knowledge-

generating one. In these models, science should not stand outside society, but should acknowledge that it is inextricably bound up with the social order, and be striving to improve that social order (that is, research *shouldn't* be value-free).

A rejection of the 'value-free' aims of research is central to the *critical tradition* in social research, which Lee Harvey described as having the following elements:

> [The critical tradition] regards the positivistic scientific method as unsatisfactory because it deals only with surface appearances. Instead, critical social research methodology cuts through surface appearance. It does so by locating social phenomena in their specific historical context ... within a prevailing social structure. Critical social research analyses this structure ... and its ideological manifestations and processes. ... Critical social research includes an overt political struggle against oppressive social structures. (Harvey 1990: 19–20)

For Harvey, the distinguishing element of critical methodology is that epistemology and critique are intertwined: there can be no pure knowledge, and the task of methodology is to unpack the status of knowledge, and the processes by which it comes to be accepted. This perspective covers a number of traditions in the social sciences. Here we introduce two of them, feminist and participatory approaches, which have had a significant impact on the development of qualitative methodology in terms of positing rather different goals from the traditional ones of value-free inquiry, and have both been influential in the field of health.

Feminist approaches

The advent of 'second wave' feminist activism in the late 1960s has been mirrored by the development of feminist theory and research both within and outside the academy. This was notable in that it highlighted the relationship between knowledge and power, not just that knowledge enables empowerment but that the legitimation of knowledge claims is tied to social structures of domination. To this end, feminist theorists demonstrated that what counted as 'knowledge' reflected a masculine world-view – for example, reflecting only male experiences or concerns. Underlying this perspective is a notion of *difference*, whether it was to claim that men and women are *essentially* different (i.e. that, to some extent, biology is destiny) or that men and women occupy different *social* positions and therefore have very different world-views and experiences. This caused the claims of natural science to objectivity to be called into question. If knowledge supposedly mirrors an independently existing world, how do we account for the different subjectivities of women and men? This led to the development of the feminist 'standpoint theorists'. These included Sandra Harding (1986), who argued that all knowledge is produced by social subjects, and knowledge that is being produced predominantly by men about a world that is predicated on male experiences and views cannot be held to be objective. What this therefore implies is the need for an explicitly feminist science.

However, one of the earliest tensions within feminist theorizing arose from this. Feminism as a social movement is (in common with other social movements such as the black, gay, peace or ecological movements) an emancipatory project. It has its roots in Enlightenment ideals of justice and freedom; that is, a commitment to social change. Nonetheless, it also shares with the theories that underpin these other social movements a critique of these ideals. Notions of 'justice' and 'freedom' imply an absolute, objective existence independent of any power relations, but this becomes untenable in the face of the critique of 'objectivity' and the commitment to making the subjectivity of knowledge claims explicit. A further debate in feminist theorizing was over the principle of essentialism or relativism. This called into question the very existence of the categories 'male' and 'female'. Feminist theorists such as those of the French psychoanalytical school (see, for example, Irigaray 1985; Wittig 1992) attempted to examine the processes by which subjects came to have a gendered consciousness. Others, from more sociological traditions, such as Judith Butler (1990) and Donna Haraway (1991), have addressed the concept of gender as a social construction as part of the 'postmodern' turn in social theory.

In research terms it is clear that the particular feminist epistemological framework adopted, whether standpoint or constructionist, will determine both the research question and the subsequent research design.

Participatory approaches

Another justification for rejecting the positivist notion of striving for a value-neutral science is because one consequence of this is a consolidation of knowledge within a small elite, and an unhealthy separation of scientists from the wider society. Following on from this, researchers from participatory traditions of methodology see research as ideally a co-operative enterprise, involving working with communities as co-investigators. For some, this has liberationist aims, and the purpose of research should be to engage in dialogue with oppressed people in order to further emancipation. Peter Reason (1998) has identified three strands in participatory inquiry, which he labels co-operative inquiry, participatory action research and action inquiry. Co-operative inquiry assumes first that all actors are self-determining – in any research project, all involved are both researchers and subjects, co-operating by reflexively drawing upon their own experiences. Participatory action research is explicit about the relationship between knowledge and power, seeing the role of the researcher as liberating communities through research activities that shift the balance of knowledge. The aims are thus to produce understanding that is useful for the group you are working with, and to empower those people, rather than to do research 'on' them. Action inquiry is primarily orientated towards change, but involves a conscious approach to action, in which an organization or community develops a collaborative and reflexive awareness. Although the emancipatory aims of participatory approaches are perhaps more associated with research in developing country settings (see, for instance, Case Study 2.2, which used participatory methods as part of an evaluation of a sexual health programme in The Gambia), the collaborative and action-orientated elements of these approaches have influenced health care researchers in developed country settings as well. Julienne Meyer, for instance, has written widely on the challenges of using action research methods in nursing research in the UK (Meyer 1993, 1997) and argues that, despite challenges (such as the difficulty in integrating these methods with current frameworks of research funding), the role of action research is likely to be greater in the future, with a growing focus on interdisciplinary knowledge production and an emphasis on more 'porous' research structures that are less constrained by elitist university research and more open to partnerships with practitioners.

The orientations of qualitative research

There are, then, some very different theoretical and epistemological starting points in qualitative research, although many of them share a rejection of one or more of the elements of a positivist tradition in social science. These starting points will influence the kinds of research question that researchers address, and how they go about generating knowledge. Clearly, what counts as a 'proper' research question, and what counts as valid knowledge, will depend on macro-theoretical assumptions about the world, middle-range theories that are often rooted in specific disciplines, and epistemological assumptions. This might suggest that to talk of 'qualitative research' in general is impossible, given the plurality of perspectives researchers bring to bear on health. However, there are some broad orientations to methodology that are shared by many researchers, although not of course by all, or at all times. They are: a commitment to naturalism, a focus on understanding, and a flexible approach to research strategy.

Naturalism

'Naturalism' refers to a preference for studying phenomena in their 'natural' environment. We know that behaviour, including health behaviour, is contextual. It is, for instance, a common experience that we take more 'risks' with our health when on holiday than at home. Similarly, we are likely to behave differently while being studied than when not. This was a key finding of the famous Hawthorne studies, in which researchers found that human behaviour (in this case productivity in a factory) altered as a result of taking part in the study, rather than any of the specific interventions being tested. Rather than continuing with experimental methods, the Hawthorne researchers turned to ethnographic methods such as interviewing and observation to understand worker behaviour (see Schwartzman 1993 for a discussion). Studying health behaviour in a 'natural' environment allows us to study how, for instance, people manage medication regimes in the busy context of their everyday lives, rather than as part of a drug trial. Talking to people in depth, allowing them to tell their own story, provides us access to their world-view rather than that of the researcher. Ethnographic methods (see Chapter 6) are perhaps the most 'naturalistic' in that they attempt to generate in-depth knowledge about a setting (whether it is a small village, or a hospital ward) over time, in order to understand how and why people believe and behave as they do. The aim is for the researcher to become part of the setting for long enough to minimize their impact.

For some social scientists, it is 'naturalism' that defines a distinct qualitative methodological approach, and separates it from the methods of inquiry used in the natural sciences. Norman Denzin (1971), for instance, uses the term 'naturalistic behaviourism' to describe an empirical approach to studying the social world, with its own logic. For Denzin, social research should be closely tied to the everyday, routine lives of the people researched, aiming to understand their perspective and then 'reproduce in a rich and detailed fashion the experiences, thoughts and languages' of those studied. What distinguishes this enterprise from common-sense accounts of the same world is that the researcher 'attempts to impose order on the social world'. Naturalistic research is not merely the production of detailed, empathetic accounts of social worlds such as those of a hospital clinic or small village, but the theoretical analysis of them.

'Naturalism' is of course an idealistic notion, as there is in practice no 'untainted' research field observable by the researcher. Any act of observation will impact on the field, however 'invisible' the researcher becomes, and the researcher needs a reflexive approach that takes into account their interrelationship with the field studied. However, an orientation towards naturalism means that the qualitative researcher is more likely to be interested in the everyday, or 'real life', context than in ideal situations, and is more likely to explicitly reflect on how the research setting has in itself had an impact on behaviour.

A focus on meaning and understanding

Following on from the interpretative tradition in the social sciences, much qualitative research focuses on understanding the world from the point of view of the participants in the study. The starting assumption is often perhaps a generous one: that most people, most of the time, are rational and sensible in their choices if we can understand the constraints they are under, what their priorities are, and what they are trying to achieve. As the American sociologist Erving Goffman (1961), who studied behaviour in psychiatric hospitals, put it:

> any group of persons . . . develop a life of their own that becomes meaningful, reasonable and normal once you get close to it . . . a good way to learn about any of these worlds is to

submit oneself in the company of the members to the daily round of petty contingencies to which they are subject. (Goffman 1961: ix–x)

Thus, the best qualitative research starts by asking not what people get wrong, or don't know, or why they behave irrationally, but instead seeks to identify what they *do* know, how they maintain their health, and what the underlying rationality of their behaviour is. In the example in Case Study 1.1, for instance, apparently irrational behaviour (not taking medication as prescribed for a potentially disabling disease) becomes understandable if we see it from the point of view of those diagnosed with asthma. This is equally true of research with health workers. Doctors who refuse to implement evidence-based guidelines or nurses who don't wash their hands between caring for different patients are unlikely to be acting merely ignorantly or 'irrationally', and the aim of a qualitative study on their behaviour should be to focus on what they are achieving, and how, rather than what they are not doing, and why. Qualitative research attempts to understand the world (or the part of it we are interested in) from the perspective of the participant, not the researcher. So the most productive question may not necessarily be 'Why don't doctors implement evidence-based guidelines?' but 'How do doctors use evidence-based guidelines? What kind of evidence is used in their work? How are guidelines integrated into the day-to-day work doctors have to accomplish?'

The benefits of this orientation towards understanding for health research are clear. Public health and health promotion, for instance, are often concerned with changing behaviour. Without an empathetic understanding of why people behave as they do, we are unlikely to identify the possibilities for change.

Flexible research strategies

In carrying out a large-scale survey or an epidemiological study, it is usual to plan most of the research in detail before beginning, including the sample size, the precise data to be collected, and the statistical tests likely to be used in analysis. Although qualitative studies also need careful planning, it is more common to have a flexible research strategy, which can be adapted as early data are produced and analysed. As a model it may be helpful to divide up the research process into stages such as literature review, research design, data collection, analysis and writing up, but in practice these stages are much more likely to overlap in qualitative work, and will inform each other. Early data analysis may suggest, for instance, a more refined (or even completely different) research question that will influence later sampling, and may send you back to look for more literature. As we shall see in Chapter 10, the process of writing up is an essential part of the analysis in most qualitative work.

The degree of flexibility required depends on the demands of the study and the perspective of the researcher. In some studies, flexibility may mean simply adding to the intended sample in order to add more depth to one finding. In others, the research design is developed as the study continues, utilizing a number of different methods and approaches as the researcher unearths new clues to the answers they are seeking. One metaphor that is sometimes used to describe the qualitative researcher in this approach is the French term 'bricoleur' (Lévi-Strauss 1966) or professional 'do-it-yourself' person. This is a kind of skilled Jack or Jill of all trades, who can utilize, adapt and devise methods of inquiry and bodies of literature as the need arises throughout a project (Denzin and Lincoln 1998). This approach has great appeal in health research, where so many aspects of everyday life impinge on the topic of interest, and we are often required to shift perspectives throughout a project, or utilize unexpected opportunities for data collection. It may, however, be difficult to pursue in funded research, with most sponsors wanting clear protocols at the outset of a study.

Added to naturalism, interpretation and flexibility, Bryman suggested two other characteristics of qualitative approaches: description and process (Bryman 1988: 63–6). By 'description' he meant a tendency towards detailed (or 'thick') description, rather than a focus on explanation. Detailed description allows the broader context of social behaviours to be delineated. Following from the emphasis on context in qualitative research, Bryman argued, is an emphasis on process. This, he believes, is both a consequence of an orientation towards wanting (historical) context and a reflection of an underlying belief that participants perceive the world as an unfolding sequence of changes, so research should capture this. Qualitative studies therefore emphasize the processes underpinning social activity through detailed descriptions of the participants' behaviours, beliefs, and the contexts within which they occur.

Together with the epistemological traditions outlined above, these orientations towards naturalism, understanding and flexibility imply some other common assumptions that qualitative researchers work with. The recognition of the contextual nature of knowledge and behaviour, and an emphasis on understanding, implies an acceptance of different world-views. In studying the organization of a rural clinic, we should not be surprised if the accounts given by patients and nurses are very different. It is not that one group is misinformed or mistaken, but that each provides an account that is rooted in different worlds. The task of the researcher is not to adjudicate between competing accounts, or to undermine the 'truth' of one, but to understand, from the perspective of those participants, how the world is the way they describe it. This is not an easy task, particularly when researching topics that are close to the researcher's own professional experience.

A second implication is that qualitative research is properly sceptical of received wisdom; that is, common-sense accounts and assumptions, whether these are from academics or participants in the field. Treating an account of clinic organization from a nurse as a valid account, given his or her perspective, is not the same as treating this as the 'truth' about clinic organization. The researcher is not merely a reporter, taking down stories from the field to report back. They must also analyse those accounts, and link the empirical findings with a theoretical understanding of health care organizations, of nursing work, or of professional–client encounters. Equally, the 'common sense' of health care knowledge must be questioned. Qualitative research properly questions the categories it is presented with, rejecting the normative assumptions built into many research studies. Thus, in studying the introduction of 'patient-centred care' to a ward, we should be careful not to assume that 'patient-centred care' is inevitably a good thing, or that it means the same thing to different actors. In studying the 'barriers to evidence-based practice', it is important to remember that these are only likely to be 'barriers' from the perspective of advocates of evidence-based practice.

The contribution of qualitative research to understanding health and health services

Finally, this chapter considers a question that, even if qualitative researchers do not ask themselves, may be asked of them by others: what are the results of a qualitative study likely to contribute to policy or practice? The examples throughout this book illustrate some of the contributions that qualitative research findings have made to professional practices in areas such as public health, health promotion, health service planning and policy. Qualitative researchers are often called on to 'defend' their methods, particularly if they work in settings where these approaches have not been seen as posing legitimate questions or 'scientific' ways of answering them. There are, perhaps, three broad approaches to answering this kind of criticism.

The first is to appeal to the 'deficit model' of traditional clinical and epidemiological research, and argue that qualitative methods 'reach the parts other methods can't reach'. Thus, Green and Britten (1998) argue that qualitative research has a potential role in contributing to the 'evidence base' of medicine because it can answer questions that experimental methods cannot address, such as the meaning of medication for patients, the social processes by which 'evidence' is utilized, or the interactional processes at work in the health care consultation. Thus, the deficit model suggests that the specific contribution of qualitative methods to public health lies in their ability to answer important questions that cannot be answered from a quantitative perspective. Case Study 1.2, an example of how qualitative methods are used in an evaluation, illustrates this. Here, qualitative methods are needed to answer questions about process and the meaning of interventions for those providing and receiving them: they answer questions that cannot be addressed by the quantitative evaluation.

A second potential response is to appeal to the epistemological positions outlined above. Questions in qualitative work are largely about *understanding* different perspectives, or examining how reality is constructed, rather than explaining one 'reality'. Qualitative designs thus provide 'better' answers to

---

Case Study 1.2   Evaluating an intervention to improve TB care in South Africa

(Source: Lewin, S., Daniels, K., Dick, J., Zwarenstein, M. and van der Walt, H. (2002) *A qualitative evaluation of the Kopana TB training intervention.* Internal Report, Health Systems Research Unit, Medical Research Council of South Africa)

Cape Town, South Africa, has high rates of tuberculosis (TB) and clinics face problems in persuading patients to complete the long course of therapy needed to cure it and bring the epidemic under control. Previous research suggested that one barrier to patient compliance could be poor support from staff, who have a 'task orientation', rather than patient orientation, to their work. The Kopana project aimed to deliver a participative, experiential training intervention to clinic staff that would lead to improved communication with patients through patient-centred care and an orientation towards quality improvement. An experimental design, in which clinics were randomly allocated to either receive or not receive the Kopana training package, was used to evaluate the intervention. This used quantitative measures, including TB treatment completion rates, to look at the effectiveness of the intervention, and a qualitative evaluation to look at the process. The aims of the qualitative evaluation were to explore how the intervention was developed and implemented, and what impacts it had on staff, clinic organization and patients.

Simon Lewin and colleagues used ethnographic approaches to study the process of training and its impact on clinic organization. This included observations of TB clinic routines and the Kopana training sessions, interviews with staff, and analysis of transcripts of the training sessions. The findings from this ethnographic study first helped identify why Kopana did not have the anticipated outcomes; that is, it did not reduce TB cure rates significantly in the intervention clinics. A key reason was that in many clinics what the researchers call the 'integrity of the intervention' was difficult to maintain. For various logistic and organizational reasons, it was impossible to deliver the training package (which involved six facilitated sessions with clinic staff leading up to them identifying changes in practice, plus a follow-up session) in line with intention. This is perhaps typical of training interventions: although they may work well with enthusiastic advocates in initial projects, when rolled out as realistic interventions in randomly chosen settings, they are resisted and adapted by recipients in unpredictable ways. Other findings from the qualitative evaluation were that 'task orientation' was deeply entrenched as a pattern of provision in this setting, and was hard to shift through the process of Kopana training; that lack of middle management involvement may inhibit change; and that extensive health system restructuring at the same time as the intervention had created uncertainty among clinic staff and a high rate of turnover of experienced nurses. Qualitative interviews enable the researchers to look in detail at staff concerns. In some clinics, staff fears about local gangsters causing trouble in the waiting rooms, or worries about catching TB themselves, meant that an intervention designed to increase patient-centred care raised concerns about reducing the amount of control they had over patients. In others, deep-seated interpersonal conflicts between staff members or inadequate management limited the impact of any intervention that relied on building on team-working. Nurses did not necessarily identify themselves as part of a clinic team, so an intervention addressing 'the team' did not resonate with their perspectives.

The qualitative study therefore helped unpack the results of the quantitative evaluation, in explaining why the intended outcomes had not occurred. It also suggested some issues to consider in future attempts to change the delivery of care for TB patients in primary level clinics. The ethnographic study also produced findings of wider significance, given the paucity of data on the organization of care in settings such as this one. Detailed accounts of how clinic organization is achieved from the perspective of staff involved, and why apparently irrational organization structures (such as 'task orientation') persist, are useful for building future interventions that take account of the motivations and behaviour of staff, rather than making assumptions about why nurses act in the way they do.

questions located in less positivist epistemologies. Nick Black (1994), for instance, cites a study of doctors' views of audit. Although most surveys suggested that doctors were in favour of audit, observation showed that little was carried out. A qualitative study identified a raft of reasons why doctors were uncertain or even unsupportive of audit, few of which had been raised in surveys. Designs that maximize access to these different perspectives are more likely to generate useful information for policy-making than those that merely ask for respondents' views in an unsophisticated way. Qualitative methodologies, then, can be presented as generating 'better' data on beliefs and behaviour.

The third approach is a pragmatic one that cites the 'usefulness' of qualitative findings at practice and policy levels. For individual professionals, qualitative findings are often useful for 'sensitizing' them to patients' views. In Case Study 1.1, for instance, several possible orientations towards asthma medication are described. It is less important to quantify what proportion of the population would share these views than to sensitize professionals to these as possible viewpoints. The 'usefulness' of this study lies in part in its potential to alert practitioners to possible patient perspectives, and how they affect health behaviour. At the policy level, qualitative studies have the potential to provide evidence for population needs, the development of appropriate policy, and evidence for how to implement policy with health care staff. To return to the examples of qualitative health research studies given in Box 1.1, looking at the conclusions of the studies listed illustrates what their contributions to policy or practice might be:

- The study of the impact of guinea worm disease identified a 'strong co-operative ethic' among the women in the communities, which could be utilized in guinea worm prevention strategies (Watts et al. 1989).
- Understanding why cancer patients may not want information at particular times helps inform a national cancer information strategy that is based on understanding patients' needs, rather than common-sense assumptions about patients' needs (Leydon et al. 2000).
- Interviewing those seeking health information on the Internet demonstrated some benefits for users: the ability to ask embarrassing questions, information about a wide range of health provisions, and access to information that could then be discussed with their doctor. Understanding how people use health information provides guidance for those interested in providing information for the public on the Internet (Hardey 1999).
- An ethnographic study of Limba views about leprosy was used to evaluate the effectiveness of a leprosy control programme and to aid communication between health professionals and their patients, as both groups had misunderstandings about the beliefs of the other (Opala and Boillot 1996).
- The study of parents' views about the MMR vaccine found that parents felt more information from health professionals, shared in an open manner, would have helped their decisions and concluded 'only by fully appreciating the concerns of parents will health professionals be able to ... restore their confidence in the MMR' (Evans et al. 2001).

Conclusion

Qualitative health research in general, then, aims to answer 'what', 'how' or 'why' questions about social aspects of health, illness and health care. Although the contribution of qualitative research to our understanding of such activities as health behaviour and health provision is now broadly welcomed, qualitative researchers do still face some scepticism from those rooted in other research traditions. We have suggested this arises in part from differences in epistemological assumptions, with the preference for non-positivist approaches in qualitative methodology. We have also suggested the range of approaches covered by qualitative methodology, including interpretative, constructionist and critical traditions. Whilst these approaches generate different research questions, there are perhaps some shared perspectives, including preferences for naturalistic studies, a focus on meaning, and flexible research strategies.

KEY POINTS
- Research questions arise from particular theoretical frameworks.
- Most qualitative research rejects a positivist epistemology, and instead adopts interpretative, constructionist or critical methodological approaches.
- Qualitative methodologies often adopt the perspectives of naturalism, a focus on meaning and understanding and flexible research strategies.

EXERCISE

Look at the abstracts of qualitative health research papers in a social science or biomedical journal. Identify any theoretical assumptions made by the authors, either explicitly or implicitly. What other theoretical frameworks could have been used to address the topic?

FURTHER READING

Pope, C. and Mays, N. (2000) *Qualitative research in health care* (2nd ed.) London: BMJ Books. A very useful introductory reader, with chapters on the key methods of data collection and analysis.

Murphy, E., Dingwall, R., Greatbatch, D., Parker, S. and Watson, P. (1998) 'Qualitative research methods in health technology assessment: a review of the literature', *Health Technology Assessment*, 2(16). Chapter 1 of this review has a good discussion of the foundations of qualitative research perspectives, the philosophical underpinnings of the main traditions in qualitative research, and a brief history of two disciplines, medical sociology and social anthropology.

2

Developing Qualitative Research Designs

CHAPTER SUMMARY

The 'logic' of developing research protocols suggests first identifying a specific research question and then developing an appropriate research design to generate data that will answer the question. Some guidelines for developing research designs in this way are suggested, and five general types of design (experimental, survey, observational, case study and action research) are described. In practice, qualitative research design is often an iterative process, with theoretical concerns shaping the kinds of questions in which a researcher is interested, and methodological preferences influencing the research design and type of data collection methods chosen. The term 'qualitative research' is also used to refer to those components of larger studies that use qualitative data collection methods, and this chapter concludes by identifying how qualitative methods are incorporated into broader programmes of health research.

Introduction

There are a number of tasks associated with research design, including refining the research question to be addressed, deciding what sort of study it will be, how the data will be identified, collected or generated, and how they will be analysed. There should be coherence between these elements such that the type of study and data collection methods chosen are capable of addressing the question. In qualitative work, research design has traditionally been very 'loose', in that the precise aims of the study may not be known at the outset, and decisions about how to collect data or what the data will be 'about' may emerge as the research progresses. Indeed, if the topic is one with little previous research, the aim may well be a purely exploratory one of identifying some interesting issues to follow up, or 'furthering our understanding' of a setting or a social group. Decisions such as what data collection methods to use, who will be included in the sample, or how long fieldwork will last may well change in the light of early fieldwork experience, and the relevant research question may only emerge in the later stages of data analysis. In Chapter 1, this kind of flexibility was identified as a characteristic of much qualitative research.

However, for most studies, whether small unfunded student projects or large programmes, you will need a research proposal or protocol early on which sets out the key elements of the study: what you want to know, how you will find out, and why. The protocol is a kind of map of the study, and will include practical considerations such as resources needed, ethical issues and time scale. This will need to be much 'tighter' than merely an outline of why a particular topic looks like an interesting one to explore. Most funders of health research, understandably, expect research protocols to demonstrate that the proposed study is both feasible and likely to produce findings useful for public health. This chapter discusses the issues researchers need to consider when developing protocols for qualitative studies.

Research questions

The first element of research design is the 'what' – the question you want to answer. It is not common to have a formal hypothesis to test in qualitative work, but this does not mean that research questions should be vague or unrefined. A research question is more than the title of the study or description of the topic you are interested in. Ideally, it frames fairly precisely what question will be answered, and identifies clearly how it will be addressed. Good research questions are 'researchable' in that they are contained and specified enough for the proposed study to produce the data to answer them. They identify the key indicators that will be used to gather empirical evidence for the concepts of interest. Refining such questions from the 'problem' or vague topic of interest is a skill that takes time to develop. The first problem for many beginning researchers is to identify a broad topic, and there are a number of ways of generating ideas. Some productive sources of potential research questions include:

- Puzzles about the social world – everyday life generates a number of puzzles about health beliefs and behaviour that give rise to potential research questions: Why are suicide rates higher for men than for women? Why do many people consult with 'alternative' practitioners in countries where biomedical care is free? How is information technology such as the Internet being used by the public?
- Professional practice may also throw up puzzles: Why does our unit have trouble recruiting enough nurses? Why don't patients take the medicines we prescribe? Why do some ward teams seem to function better than others?
- Reading the literature may reveal interesting 'gaps' in our knowledge of particular topics: We know a lot about how parents view adolescent mental health services, but how do adolescents themselves feel? Most of the research on hospital organization has been done in industrialized countries – how generalizable is it to other settings?
- Commissioned research. Sponsors, such as government departments or health authorities, propose specific questions that they want answering to inform policy development or implementation.

Ideally a researcher's curiosity and a sponsor's need coincide and there is a sponsor willing to fund your study. Turning these initial areas of interest into researchable questions is the next stage. Even when the topic has been dictated by a funding agency, there are a number of steps to take to develop a research question and identify whether that question requires a qualitative approach. One set of questions that should be considered at the beginning of the process might include:

Is this a problem that research can address?

Health care throws up daily problems for those delivering and managing it, but not all of those are research problems. If drugs are too expensive locally for most people to afford, you may not need to waste time and resources on researching the barriers to drug use, although such research is sometimes done for political gain, for instance to convince policy-makers that 'a problem' does exist. If a hospital is understaffed, dirty and overcrowded, an ethnographic study is not needed to identify the major causes of patient dissatisfaction. However, beware of 'common-sense' answers to such problems. It may be, for example, that patients are *not* particularly dissatisfied as they realize staff are delivering the best care possible in circumstances beyond their control. It may be that 'patient dissatisfaction' is related more to the attitudes of staff towards patients, or certain groups of patients, than to the material circumstances. Indeed, some of the most interesting research can arise from the questioning of taken-for-granted 'common-sense' explanations. It is perhaps particularly important not to rely on common-sense answers to 'problems' when they rely on explanations of 'ignorance', given that most people, most of the time, behave in rational ways once we understand their perspective. Case Study 2.1, on women and smoking, illustrates this; although irrational from a health perspective, Hilary Graham's (1987) study shows how smoking could be a rational coping strategy for low-income women.

Is a qualitative approach appropriate?

If you want to understand the perspectives of participants, explore the meanings they give to phenomena, or observe a process in depth, then a qualitative approach is probably appropriate. However, if there is a need for answers to questions such as 'How many people are likely to use this service over the next year?' or 'What proportion of primary care physicians prescribe this medication?', a quantitative design, or at least a quantitative element in the study, will be required. As suggested by the discussion of theory and orientations in Chapter 1, qualitative approaches are ideal for questions that require an answer about understanding participants' views, or for questions that address the meaning given to phenomena.

What are the key concepts of interest?

'Concepts' are the building blocks of theory, the 'high-level' or abstract terms in which we frame our understanding of health. These refer to macro-theoretical constructs (see Chapter 1), such as 'inequality', 'globalization', 'power', but also the middle-range theories in which our research questions are usually embedded. Here, concepts such as 'lifestyle', 'medical autonomy' or 'compliance' may be used as part of the common stock of knowledge within a particular discipline, but carry within them a set of (often implicit) assumptions.

It is worth thinking in some detail about the concepts referred to in your research study. This thinking should clarify two questions:

- First, what are the different *components* of these concepts? For something like patient 'compliance' with prescribed medication, these might include:
  - understanding the doctor's instructions;
  - collecting the prescription;
  - taking all the medicines at the time of day the doctor recommended;
  - taking the medicines in such a way as to produce the desired effect.
- Second, what are the *assumptions* you are making in using them? As Chapter 1 discussed, theoretical assumptions are always made in research, whether explicit or not, and it is worth unpacking those that frame your particular question. The notion of 'compliance' implies a number of assumptions about patients and professionals: that, for instance, professionals are the 'experts' in the partnership; that not taking medications as prescribed is a 'problem'; that it is *non-compliance* that must be explained (rather than why patients *do* take medicines in line with professionals' advice).

Case Study 2.1 Using interviews and diaries to elaborate the meaning of statistical data on women and smoking

(Source: Graham, H. (1987) 'Women's smoking and family health', *Social Science and Medicine*, 25: 47–56)

Survey evidence suggests that those women in Britain most likely to smoke are on low incomes, with children but no work outside the home. At a superficial level, this is a surprising finding, as these are the women least able to afford cigarettes and most likely to want to make lifestyle changes to promote their own and their children's health. There is also good evidence that most of the population accepts the links between smoking and poor health: lack of knowledge is unlikely to explain the prevalence of smoking in this group.

Hilary Graham designed a study to explore these findings in the context of the 'everyday world of informal health behaviour'; that is, the day-to-day routines of housework and child care with which women were engaged. Her aim was a qualitative one, to explore these worlds 'through the eyes of the mothers', and she sampled a group of low-income and single parents. To collect data on daily experiences, she first conducted interviews, but found that these provided only a snapshot of women's lives. The focus on the women's own perspective also made it difficult to gather precise information on the details of everyday life, which Graham saw as essential for providing the context of health behaviour. To collect this fine-grained detail, she also asked participants to complete a 24-hour diary, with space to record their main and other activities over the day, and presence of others.

There were important differences in the data from the interviews and the diaries. One was that smoking was significantly under-reported in the diaries, compared with interviews: in the diaries it was reported only if it was the 'main activity' at the time. Typically, only those cigarettes that marked significant breaks in the daily routines of housework and caring were reported. Graham suggests that cigarettes were the one luxury many low-income women could afford, and that they played an important role in reducing stress and structuring the daily round of caring and housework. Having a cigarette was one way to claim some 'adult time' in the context of a busy life looking after young children, and could be a legitimate way of generating some physical space away for a short time. Thus, what appeared to be irrational behaviour (spending money on smoking when it potentially damages the health of yourself and children) was comprehensible when seen in the context of women's everyday lives.

Here, the study design is essentially a qualitative one (of exploring the meaning of health behaviour from the perspective of women themselves, in the context of their everyday lives), used to shed light on a relationship between two variables (poverty and smoking) found in the quantitative data. Within her study, Graham uses a mixed method approach to collect the data. This has the advantage of providing different perspectives on the topic of interest (smoking behaviour), and the different findings play an important role in the analysis in alerting her to the meaning of cigarettes in these women's lives.

Thinking about these assumptions can help clarify early on some of the potential limitations in your research design, particularly if the 'assumptions' of those you are researching are not the same as yours. Once you have identified the assumptions built into your research question, it can be a useful exercise to identify alternatives, and frame questions in terms of those. For instance, if we have identified an assumption that 'non-compliance' with medication is a problem in the question 'Why don't patients comply with medications?', we can turn the research question round as 'Why *do* some patients comply with medication?' Even if it is not a perspective you (as a practitioner or a researcher) share, it might turn out to be a more useful way of producing knowledge about patient behaviour than exploring non-compliance.

Refining indicators for these concepts

Abstract or theoretical concepts are good for thinking with, but need refining for use in empirical research (that is, research that relies on primary data being collected or generated). It is impossible to go into the field and 'see' or record compliance, or globalization, or medical autonomy. Once the components of each concept have been identified, *indicators* can be developed for those that are crucial to the research question. Indicators are events or phenomena that reflect (or provide evidence of) components of the underlying concept of interest. These indicators need to be empirical, in that we can generate data that capture them. In quantitative work, this process is perhaps more obvious than for qualitative. If, for instance, we are interested in measuring the health status of a given population, it is possible to specify some relevant components of health (perhaps including self-reported health status, or blood pressure) and then identify researchable indicators (questionnaire items asking for self-reports, sphygmomanometer readings) that can be used to 'measure' these in the field.

The concepts used in qualitative work are often less easily 'measurable', and indeed the aim of the research may well be to 'unpack' the concept, to further our understanding of it, rather than to pin down components for measurement. Suppose the researcher is addressing the topic of 'clinical autonomy in surgical wards'. Part of the research question might involve *identifying* the components of clinical autonomy, so it is difficult to define at the outset what the research will look for. However, the work of thinking through the assumptions embedded in the research is still vital. Here, we would be interested in identifying the components of the rather nebulous concept of 'autonomy': Does it include control over treatment decisions? Control over the decision to admit patients? Responsibility for the work of other professionals? Once these components have been delineated, it is possible to think about how the research might generate empirical evidence for them, for instance by looking specifically at how clinical decisions are made on the ward.

Refining indicators helps specify what questions the research can and can't answer. Take the example of compliance again. If we have identified 'taking the medicines at the time of day recommended by the doctor' as one component, we can then think about what would constitute evidence for that. Observation of behaviour (watching patients to see when they took medicines) might provide good evidence, but of course is unlikely to be feasible, and anyway would only provide evidence of what happened when a researcher was watching. More feasible possibilities might include asking patients to complete a diary each day, noting when they took their medicines, or interviewing them, and asking for self-reports of when medicines were taken. Neither of these are particularly good indicators for the *behaviour* of taking medicine, as they are really evidence of patients' records of that behaviour, or patients' accounts of that behaviour. The research question would have to reflect this, perhaps asking 'How do patients report compliance?' A key element in refining indicators for qualitative studies is, then, to pay careful attention to the method of data collection and to make sure the data generated by the proposed study are capable of reflecting these indicators.

Defining a research question

The different theoretical starting points outlined in Chapter 1 clearly shape the way in which researchers frame research questions, and which kinds of questions they are drawn to in the first place (see Box 1.2 in Chapter 1). These are often implicit, in that the reports of the research may not refer to them, but they nonetheless influence the kinds of issues or problems in which researchers are interested and how they turn them into research questions. It is worth asking yourself right at the beginning of a project which theoretical frame is implicit in your research question and then deliberately considering how alternative perspectives might have generated different questions, different types of information (data) needed to answer the question, and different ways of acquiring that information (data collection methods).

As an example from Box 1.2 in Chapter 1, on different possible approaches to researching the topic of immunization, if we wanted to address the question 'What sources of knowledge do parents draw on to assess the risks of immunization?', we might want to refine that in the light of a discussion about the components of 'sources of knowledge' and 'risks', and how we might identify evidence of these (indicators). We would need, for instance, to consider what would be evidence of 'drawing on a source of knowledge'. Suppose one potential source of knowledge was a newspaper report. Potential kinds of evidence for different components of this might include: mentioning newspapers unprompted in an interview about immunizations; saying 'yes' to a direct question about whether this was a source of knowledge; and using citations of newspaper reports in everyday conversation with others as a way of legitimizing beliefs about immunization risks. These kinds of evidence will imply different data generation methods (in-depth interviews, survey interviews, and perhaps focus groups or observation, respectively). The next step is then a balancing act between what is needed to answer the original question and what is feasible. One outcome might be a study that used interviews with parents, asking them about their views of immunization risks and asking directly about how they have come to know about these risks. The research question might then be refined as: 'How do parents account for their knowledge of immunization risks in interviews?'

The aim of refining the research question is, then, to generate a feasible question that it is possible to answer with the methods proposed and within the resources available. Inevitably this involves a number of 'trade-offs'. There is no 'perfect' design, and in refining the research question, most researchers have to leave out some components of interest to ensure that the study is feasible, or accept that the data generated may not provide a complete answer.

Research designs: some examples

Research design refers to the logic of the study: the what, how and why of data production. It will include the type of study proposed (such as an experiment or a case study) and the intended methods of producing data (such as interviews or observation). Clearly, the design should be appropriate to the research question. This sounds obvious, but many (even published) studies progress with a design that cannot possibly answer the proposed question. This may be because of inadequate work at the design stage, or because resource restrictions limit the scope of the study. The research design, and therefore the question, may, then, have to be tailored to meet resources. There are many ways of classifying research designs. Some take the experiment as the ideal, or prototype, research design and describe others in terms of how they resemble an experiment. Most qualitative researchers take a rather different starting point in selecting an appropriate design, and begin by considering the kind of data that will be generated. Those trained in ethnographic methods, for instance, may begin by thinking about what kinds of questions these methods might help them address in a given setting. The following list is, therefore, not a definitive typology of all research designs, but rather suggestive of the kinds of design you are likely to come across in health research.

Experiments

An experiment is perhaps the 'classic' design of the positivist tradition, as it sets up a study capable of answering a question about cause and effect. Essentially, an experiment involves an intervention, with observations before and after to identify the effect of that intervention. Ideally, experiments should have a 'control' group, who do not receive the intervention, as well as an 'intervention' group who do, to allow the researcher to separate those changes that would have happened anyway from those resulting from the intervention. Figure 2.1 illustrates the logic of experimental research design. This is perhaps a design most familiar in the natural sciences, but qualitative methods are sometimes used within experimental designs. In medical sciences, the 'rando-

Measurements at time 1	Intervention?	Measurements at time 2
Experimental group	✓	Experimental group
Control group	×	Control group

Figure 2.1   *The logic of experimental research design.*

mized controlled trial' (RCT) is considered the 'gold standard' design for testing interventions. This kind of experiment randomly allocates participants to the control and intervention group, to eliminate bias from differences between the two groups. RCTs are used extensively in trials of new medicines, where it is important to identify precisely what the effect of the intervention is. However, there has been recent interest in extending this kind of methodology to complex health service interventions, such as training schemes for staff, or new modes of treatment delivery. In these studies, sometimes called 'pragmatic trials' to suggest that they are testing 'real world' effects, qualitative methods may be used to generate data from 'before' and 'after' the intervention.

One example is Ann Oakley's (1990) evaluation of an intervention designed to increase support for new mothers. She used in-depth interviews in an experiment designed to evaluate whether social support in pregnancy (provided by research midwives) had an impact on outcomes such as mothers' satisfaction with care and infant birth weight. Oakley makes a strong argument for using experiments more widely in health research, given that they are the most appropriate design for evaluating interventions, and produce the strongest evidence for policy-makers. She also notes many of the problems facing those trying to implement pragmatic trials in health service settings. First, front-line staff may be very resistant to the process of randomization. Professional ideologies stress the value of offering services based on need, and allocating services randomly may seem perverse to practitioners, especially if some clients are apparently in greater need, or the professionals have strong feelings about the worth of the intervention. Much work is needed to demonstrate that there is genuine uncertainty about whether clients would benefit from the intervention or not. Second, the process of gaining informed consent from participants needs considerable thought. If consent is to be truly 'informed', then the trial risks being 'contaminated' by those allocated to the control group attempting to gain support from outside the trial. Another example of the use of qualitative methods to evaluate an intervention with an experimental design was described in Case Study 1.2.

In summary, experimental designs are the strongest ones for demonstrating cause and effect relationships, and thus for evaluating the effect of interventions. Qualitative methods can have a role in studying the process of trial implementation and in collecting the data needed. However, few qualitative studies utilize an experimental design because the aims of qualitative methodology are usually around understanding or interpretation, rather than determining cause and effect relationships.

Surveys

Survey is the general term for a design that aims to collect the same set of data for every 'case' in the study. Classic surveys include censuses of the population, which collect a set of information about every person in the country. More usually, health researchers will use *sample surveys*, which collect a set of data from a sample of the whole population of interest. Surveys are the design of choice for descriptive quantitative research questions (how many people in the locality need this service, or have had this kind of experience?), or when we want to look for associations between two measurable variables, such as health care experiences and demographic characteristics. Although we usually think of quantitative data when we think of surveys, in which questionnaires or structured interviews are used to collect information, many interview studies utilize survey designs. The study in Case Study 1.1, in which the researchers interviewed people about their asthma, can be thought of as a survey design, in that a similar set of data (beliefs about asthma, use of medication, demographic details) has been collected for all of those interviewed. However, the aim of this study was not to study the interviewees as a sample of the whole population of asthma patients, or to look for statistical associations between the variables, but a rather more qualitative one of looking at patient narratives.

To some extent, the logic of experimental and survey design is rooted in a positivist epistemology, in which the aim of research is explanation, and there is an assumption that, ideally, a stable 'truth' about the world (whether causal relationships or descriptions of population) can be discovered. Not all research questions are about cause and effect and, following from the orientations outlined above, many studies begin with quite different aims – to understand the social world, rather than to explain it. The remaining designs are more rooted in a qualitative style of research, rather than those that just use qualitative methods within other designs.

Observational studies

If the aims of the research are describing and understanding what is going on in a particular social setting, then observational designs are called for, which allow the researcher to document social life in its 'natural' state. Many qualitative studies utilize the logic of observational design, in that they aim to document everyday life, or explore some aspect of life in its 'natural' context. Observational designs include ethnographic studies that aim to provide a rich, 'thick' description of a particular setting, and studies of naturally occurring data such as videos of health service consultations. These are described in Chapter 6. The key characteristic of an observational design is that the researcher does not intervene (or at least not deliberately) and seeks instead to document what happens in everyday contexts, rather than research ones. The 'data' are thus the naturally occurring talk and behaviour of those being studied. Examples of observational studies include Rosenhan's study of psychiatric hospitals described in Case Study 3.2, in which researchers became patients to observe hospital admission procedures and routines, and the study summarized in Case Study 6.2, which utilized tape recordings of consultations between doctors and their patients.

Case studies

For some writers on methods, describing a study as a 'case study' merely identifies the way in which the sample for the study is selected (Hammersley 1992a) or the data reported (Wolcott 2002). Martyn Hammersley (1992a: 184), for example, defines a case study as research investigating a small number of naturally occurring cases, as opposed to an experiment (in which the cases are created by the researcher) or a survey (in which a large number of cases are investigated). For Hammersley, there is no specific logic implied by a 'case study', nor do they have any specific theoretical or methodological characteristics, so we should not define it as a type of design. In this view, selecting a case study design rather than a survey or experiment involves decisions about what the aims of the sample are. If the need is for empirical generalizability, then a survey will be appropriate; if depth and accuracy are needed, a case study will be. If the need is for evidence of causal relationships, an experiment will be preferable; if we want to examine naturally occurring rather than artificial phenomena, then a case study will have advantages.

However, others have argued that case studies represent a distinctive research design and methodological approach, with implications beyond those of sample selection. Robert Yin (1994) argues that the case study is the research design of choice when 'a "how" or "why" question is being asked about a contemporary set of events over which the investigator has little control' (Yin 1994: 9). A case study involves studying a phenomenon (such as a change in health service management structures, or health practices of rural villagers) within its context (the hospital, the village). Yin distinguishes case studies from other designs by noting that they explicitly include context, unlike experiments (which attempt to 'control out' context) and surveys (which can only include the context considered at the outset, when designing the questionnaire). Classic case studies include traditional ethnographies, in which the researcher spends many months, or years, in one 'field' and aims to write an in-depth account of the community (see Chapter 6). They typically involve a combination of data collection methods, such as observation, documentary analysis and interviews.

One particular type of case study is the *life history*, based on the story of one individual. Ken Plummer (1983) sees the life history as acting as a 'humanist' corrective to the more positivist and generalizing traditions in the social sciences, through its focus on individuality, subjectivity and the particular.

Although perhaps not widely used in health research, there are some interesting examples from the literature that illustrate the potential of this approach. Plummer cites life stories collected from heroin addicts, a woman dying of terminal cancer, and prostitutes, which could all be used to provide an individual perspective on policy issues, some insight into change over time and, in many cases, invaluable information about the impact of social structures on individuals that could not be accessed in any other way. One illustration from the health field is Pauline Prior's (1995) case study of a man, 'Samuel', who spent forty years as a resident of a large mental hospital in Northern Ireland. Using an analysis of case notes and interviews with professionals, Prior used Samuel's life history to illuminate changes in mental health policy and the impact of institutionalization on individuals. Despite his residence in a long-term institution, Samuel maintained a strong self-identity, and resisted a stigmatized identity as 'mentally ill' and isolated, partly, Prior argues, through his involvement in the local church and as a reliable manual worker. Drawing on theoretical perspectives on the impact of institutions on self-identity, stigmatization and deviance, Prior shows how this life history is an 'atypical' case, which can develop our understanding of institutions through exploring how some individuals resist the effects of institutionalization.

Action research

Action research, a term that is increasingly used in health research, has different meanings among its many exponents but is often rooted in a participatory approach (see Chapter 1). The distinctive element of action research design is that the research aims to *change* practice as well as studying it. The aims may not be as explicit as 'emancipation', but rather a more open and equal relationship with research participants, who have a role in setting the research agenda and contributing to design. Action research has a history in community development projects, where research questions arise clearly from social problems, such as poverty, drug use or social exclusion. In developed countries, nursing professionals in particular have seen action research as allowing researchers to address the power relationships inherent in many other research designs (Meyer 1997), and as addressing problems that arise from professional practice, rather than those imposed from outside. Hart and Bond (1995) discuss the potential of these strategies for front-line health professionals interested in improving practice or changing organizations. Rather than engaging in research with the aim of changing practice in the future, action research combines the production of knowledge with the process of changing practice. It is problem-orientated and research, action and evaluation are linked within one process. Findings are shared with participants throughout the process of the study, so that discussion can inform the subsequent stages. This leads to a cyclical research design in which planning, observing and reflecting feed back into the next planning cycle. Thus the core research topic may throw up many other issues for participants, as reflection on findings generates new questions. One criticism of action research has been the difficulty of balancing the two aims of changing practice and contributing to theory, with many reports of action research studies perhaps weak on how their findings have contributed to knowledge in the area. Case Study 2.2 (Paine et al. 2002) used an 'action research' design in developing a sexual health programme in The Gambia.

Problems with design typologies

The typology of research designs outlined above suggests the difficulties faced in attempting to classify designs. First, the divisions between different designs are not clear-cut. An 'ethnography', for instance, could be described as being an observational design or a case study. Second, it is impossible to develop an exhaustive typology – there are some studies that do not quite 'fit' any of the descriptions of designs above. Indeed, the typical qualitative health research study is often an in-depth interview study based on a small sample. Many of the case studies in this book draw on this kind of data (see, for instance, Case Studies 1.1, 2.1, 4.1, 4.2, 5.1, 5.2, 8.1 and 8.2). The 'design' of a small-scale interview study is perhaps midway between an observational study and a survey. The small-scale interview study does depend to some extent on the logic of observational work, in that the aims are often to access the 'everyday' knowledge or talk of interviewees, although of course there are limits to how far a research interview can capture naturalistic talk, as is discussed in Chapter 4. Although qualitative interviews do not aim to collect exactly the same set of data from each respondent, there are also elements of survey logic, in that the analysis might look for regularities and typologies within the interview accounts (see Chapter 8). It would be difficult to argue, though, that the interview study constitutes a separate design: there is nothing specific about the logic by which it addresses a research question, as this borrows from both the naturalism of observational designs and the format of the survey.

Most importantly, this discussion of research design in terms of logic and aim demonstrates that there is *no necessary relationship between the design of the study and the methods of data collection*. Although quantitative methods may be more associated with surveys and experiments, and qualitative with observational and case study research, this is not always the case. Oakley's experimental study of the impact of social support on pregnancy outcomes used interviews to collect some data on outcome measures, and a case study might use a mix of qualitative and quantitative methods of data collection. The *methods* of data collection used in a study should not be confused with the *design* of the study. Following from this, it is clear that the term 'qualitative research' is used in practice in two rather distinct ways:

- to describe the orientation and design of a study (qualitative methodology); and
- to describe the data collection methods used (qualitative methods).

Case Study 2.2   A participatory evaluation of the 'Stepping Stones' sexual health programme in The Gambia

(Source: Paine, K., Hart, G., Jawo, M., et al. (2002) ' "Before we were sleeping, now we are awake": preliminary evaluation of the Stepping Stones sexual health programme in The Gambia', *African Journal of AIDS Research*, 1: 41–52)

Stepping Stones is a programme that aims to 'enable participants to increase control of their sexual and emotional relationships' through a project involving community-level workshops that cover relationship skills as well as information on sexually transmitted diseases and condom use. It works with both men and women, and addresses their concerns as well as those of the research team. The research team aimed to evaluate the impact of Stepping Stones in two villages in The Gambia. Although HIV infection was relatively low in The Gambia, it was slightly higher in the intervention site and there were reported to be other negative consequences of sexual behaviour, such as subfertility and unwanted pregnancy. Intervention villages were chosen randomly from a list matched on the basis of key geographic and socio-demographic variables. The overall design of the study was, then, an experimental one.

The evaluation used a multi-method approach, including a participatory evaluation by the study villagers, in-depth interviews, focus group interviews, surveys of knowledge, attitudes and practices, and a monitoring of condom supplies. The participatory evaluation was based on a series of workshops (with separate groups of old and young men and women) carried out over ten weeks, which invited participants to consider broad topics (such as 'relationships') but in ways that facilitated them, rather than the research team, to set the priorities and to decide on action. An early way in which participants set the priorities was in shifting the focus away from 'family planning' to 'infertility prevention', which was in line with the community's own values.

The first workshop was used to prioritize health problems, and to decide which were the most urgent. Some of the sexual and reproductive health problems identified included: sex when the woman was unwilling, jealousy over co-wives, domestic violence and lack of financial support from husbands. The themes from the four groups (old and young men and women) were presented to the whole village. At one-year follow-up, the groups were asked what had changed as a result of the programme. In both intervention villages, participants listed better communication between wives and husbands, less domestic violence and safer sex outside marriage. The villagers reported enjoying the programme techniques, such as role plays.

The results of the interviews and surveys suggested that there were some important increases in the intervention villages in knowledge about sexually transmitted diseases, especially HIV, and how to prevent them. Collecting valid data from surveys on sexual knowledge and behaviour is a challenge, and the researchers drew extensively on interview data to determine the impact of Stepping Stones on issues such as condom use and knowledge about transmission of infection. Interviews suggested women had been empowered by the project to be more able to insist on condom use. However, one of the most significant findings for the project team was the broader change to relationships between men and women that emerged from the programme. Almost all interviewees reported a reduction in dissent between men and women, and the development of more effective strategies for discussing difficult issues without arguments.

This case study demonstrates how in practice research designs are often mixed: an experimental intervention is evaluated with a multi-method approach, utilizing a range of tools to access attitude and behaviour change. The underlying approach of the intervention and evaluation was that of 'participatory research', with the research team aiming to include participants in the programme, rather than researching 'on' them. The aims, then, are rather broader than disease reduction, and reflect a more holistic view of health including empowerment and capacity for community development.

Although this book is primarily concerned with qualitative studies in the first sense, the principles of 'good practice' of course apply equally well to qualitative components of other studies, or to the use of qualitative data collection techniques in other kinds of study. However, in practice there is often some tension between the epistemological traditions when qualitative methods are used in multi–disciplinary studies. Chapter 9 discusses some of the problems as well as possibilities of mixing methods and disciplinary approaches.

Influences on research design

In principle, then, the main influences on research design are the research question, adequately refined as a researchable question, and the aims of the study, such as assessing an intervention, exploring a process, or involving users in the research and changing practice. Theoretical perspectives, as introduced in Chapter 1, will also frame both the kinds of questions a researcher will ask and what legitimate kinds of answers can be generated. It would, however, be idealistic to assume that only these methodological concerns will influence research design. Political factors impact on what is likely to be funded, but also on what kinds of research are currently seen as worthy of public funds, how easy it will be to get findings published, and how influential the findings are going to be. There are also 'fashions' in particular methodologies, which make some kinds of study easier to fund at times than others.

Feasibility is also a constraint on designing the 'ideal' study. It is not always possible, ethically or practically, to do observational work. If we are interested in 'private' behaviour, such as sexual behaviour, we may be restricted to interview methods to collect accounts, rather than methods that would generate direct empirical evidence. Time may restrict a study to looking at documents when we would ideally like to interview people as well. Feasibility is also a function of who the researcher is, and what institutional affiliations and networks they can draw upon. These are to some extent opportunistic – a specific professional network and access to particular settings are likely to generate particular research questions, and also provide the resources to answer them. In some cases this relies on personal characteristics. Here, for example, is Lee Monaghan's description of why it was feasible for him to undertake an ethnographic study (see Chapter 6) of the risks faced by 'bouncers' (door staff in night clubs):

> As a reflexive ethnographer I know my male gender, relative youth (under 30 during the main study period) and bodily capital (muscular, weighing approximately 16½ stone at six-foot), represented resources for getting in and getting on with this study … my embodied social history consisting of lifting weights and boxing … rendered me willing and able to assume an active membership role [as a doorman]. (Monaghan 2003: 21)

Monaghan presumably developed an interest in the health risks faced by these workers in part because of his personal network of contacts, which in turn facilitated an entry to the field that would have been extremely difficult for anyone without his physical attributes or life experiences. Although this is an extreme example, practical issues of feasibility are likely to impact on most study designs, and any protocol should demonstrate that a study is practically doable with the resources (both material and personal) available.

An idealized logic?

So far, we have described the process of framing a research question and developing an appropriate research design as if it were both rational and time-ordered, constrained only by external factors such as available funding and feasibility. Although this is the way in which research studies are often written up (the author formulated a question and then decided how to collect data in the light of this), it represents an idealized and often post-hoc logic. Given the flexible and evolving nature of qualitative research design, it is possible that the precise research question will not emerge until quite late in the study. It may be that the researcher has a 'hunch' that a particular field is interesting, and that initial exploratory data analysis will generate a fruitful line of more detailed inquiry.

Jennifer Mason (1996) suggests a rather different logical order in research design, which perhaps reflects better the 'real' evolution of many qualitative study designs. She poses five questions that researchers should address in moving from a broad area of interest to a workable proposal for research. In summary they are:

- What is the nature of the phenomena that I want to investigate?
- What might represent knowledge or evidence of those phenomena?
- What broad topic is the research concerned with?
- What is the intellectual 'puzzle'?
- What is the purpose of my research? (Mason 1996)

This is an interesting approach to research design, as it highlights ontological and epistemological concerns at the outset, rather than assuming that they follow on from the research question. The 'nature of the phenomena' refers to the essence of the researcher's interests – whether it be individuals, perspectives, narratives, collectivities, cultures, order, disorder, or some other phenomenon. These, notes Mason, are located in very different social places, and presume very different assumptions about the nature of the world. Only through clarifying their own perspectives (from the range of alternatives that are available) can researchers identify what their research is really *about*. The second question relates to epistemological concerns. Once the phenomena of interest have been clarified, the researcher can identify what would represent evidence of them. The aims of the study thus come much later in the process for Mason, and can be addressed only in the light of answers to the first two questions. Her final question, on the purpose of the research, relates to both the immediate aims (such as contributing to knowledge, completing a PhD thesis, or developing a health promotion intervention) and the 'purpose' in terms of the precise research question that is to be answered.

In practice, much health research design is a circular and iterative process, involving a mixture of the idealized logic of formal research design, the more qualitative approach of Mason, and the many incremental and opportunistic decisions we make on the way. Some researchers are more comfortable with thinking through from the general (what is the big theoretical problem this research addresses?) to the specific (what research question will shed light on this theoretical problem?), whereas others are more comfortable thinking the other way round, and starting with the specific question and then thinking through the theoretical framework that may be most appropriate for making sense of the question. To some extent this is also constrained by the context of the research. For student projects, the researcher may have more leeway to think abstractly about the kinds of theoretical problems in which they are interested, and then move down to a feasible question that will contribute to our understanding of these problems. Professional researchers employed in applied settings may have to work with questions defined by other people, and work 'backwards' from these, although of course much qualitative work will end up reframing these initial questions.

For instance, in a study commissioned by a UK health authority to identify the 'problems' general practitioners in single-handed practice faced in providing good-quality care, Green (1993a, 1993b) found that in practice the general practitioners interviewed did not face 'problems'. From the perspective of the health authority, the working conditions of these doctors clearly presented them with 'problems', such as having to provide 24-hour-a-day care to their patients without colleagues with whom to share the burden, or being unable to take holidays. However, from the perspective of the doctors, these were not 'problems' but rather sources of pride in their ability to cope, and the 'problems' for them were located in what they perceived as their marginalization by the health authority. Their perceptions of 'good-quality care' were also rather different from those of both the health authority and their colleagues in larger practices, as they were more likely to stress the quality of the doctor–patient relationship than technical aspects of care such as services provided. The research question thus changed from 'What problems do single-handed GPs face in providing good-quality care?' to 'What is "good-quality care" from the perspective of single-handed GPs, and how do they provide it?'

Qualitative research design is, then, by necessity flexible, in that the research question may well shift throughout the process of doing the research, and the 'stages' of planning, fieldwork, analysis and writing up are rarely sequential. Each feeds into the others, as the concepts identified at the beginning are refined through analysing the data, and further through writing up the analysis. Designs in qualitative research are inevitably provisional to a large extent. However, this does not mean that the work involved in designing a project is redundant: developments in conceptual thinking do not happen in a vacuum, but in the context of particular questions, framed by a theoretical understanding of the problem. These need to be carefully considered at the outset.

Data collection/generation and analysis methods

The decision about which data generation and analysis methods to use can also be described as a logical one deriving from the needs of the study, but in practice most researchers are most 'comfortable' with or skilled in particular styles of data collection, whether ethnographic observation, in-depth interviewing, or less intrusive measures such as analysing documents. These preferences are likely to lead to particular kinds of research topics and questions being selected. The chapters in Part 2 of this book describe some of the possibilities and limitations of four ways of generating qualitative data (interviewing, group interviewing, observation and documentary analysis). These cover the major methods, but of course there are many variations on these and some we don't address. Particularly hard to reach groups or sensitive topic areas might require imaginative methods of collecting data. Rachel Baker and Rachel Hinton (1999), for instance, describe the use of video in a study of street children in Nepal, in which they chose activities to film and enacted sketches showing events in their everyday lives, such as rag picking and sleeping on the streets. The development of novel data collection methods may in itself be an aim of a study, in which case the researcher may not know at the planning stage how well they will work.

Practical issues

Once the fundamental questions about what the research is aiming to do, and how, have been addressed, planning can move on to the more practical questions. The main headings used in most research protocols are summarized in Box 2.1. Different organizations and funders have different formats for writing protocols, but most will require descriptions in varying detail of *what* you will do, *why* and *how*.

The 'methods' and more practical issues should follow on logically from the work described in the first part of this chapter. The data collection methods should be capable of producing the kind of information that will answer the research question, and the protocol should deal with issues of feasibility. This might include references to pilot work or discussions with collaborators to show that you can gain access to the fieldwork site, or anticipate being able to recruit the required number of interviewees. Even if the final sample size will be theoretically determined (see Chapter 4), the protocol should give some indication of likely scope, in order to cost the study. For case studies, such as ethnographies, the choice of site needs to be justified in terms of its usefulness for answering the research question.

Box 2.1 Main headings for research protocols

Aims and objectives	The 'what' of the study, including the broad aim (what you are going to do) broken down into measurable objectives
Background	The 'why': why this is an interesting question, an important question or a policy-relevant question
Methods	The 'how': a detailed description of the data you will collect and how, including sample sizes, if appropriate, and issues of access
Ethical issues	Particular ethical issues raised by your study, including whether you need and have ethical approval, and how you will address them
Resources	Costings for staff, travel and materials
Time scale	This should include important milestones, such as commencement and completion of fieldwork, draft report completion
Dissemination and outputs	How will you inform others, including participants, of the findings? What other outputs are you expecting?

Multi-method designs: the place of qualitative work in larger health research studies

Qualitative social science studies of health topics typically use one research strategy, and address a single qualitative question. However, in health research, the use of multiple methods of inquiry is becoming more common, and is encouraged by many funding bodies. This means that qualitative methods of data collection are not only used in qualitative studies. In much health research qualitative approaches are used in combination with others, or as part of a larger programme of study. For instance, the study described in Case Study 5.1 (on Bedouin views of maternal and child health) is from a larger, five-year programme of work on interventions to improve child health in the area. Case Study 1.2 is an example of qualitative research done in the context of a larger evaluation of an intervention, which included clinical outcomes as well as organizational ones. Chapter 9 discusses the issues raised by collaborative working on these kinds of multi-disciplinary programmes, but here we outline three ways in which qualitative methods might combine with other research strategies in terms of research design, either within one programme of work or as a series of studies. First, qualitative studies can be used in exploratory (or pilot) work. Here, qualitative work is logically the precursor for other designs. Second, qualitative work can follow other research, with an aim of adding 'depth' to findings from quantitative studies, or exploring the meaning of quantitative findings. Third, some projects use qualitative and other approaches in tandem, with the aim of addressing different aspects of the same research question.

Exploratory or pilot work

Qualitative work can precede quantitative work in multi-design projects for two reasons: as preparatory, or pilot, work when the aims of the proposed quantitative study are already known, or as 'hypothesis-generating' studies, in which the aims of the quantitative work will be refined when the qualitative data have been analysed.

Most projects involve some initial pilot work to look at feasibility and predict problems with implementation, and qualitative methods are often used at this point. For instance, if a large-scale trial of different treatment options was being considered, some ethnographic study of the clinical sites at which decisions were made would be sensible, to outline the possible barriers to random allocation, and the views of the staff involved. In developing a questionnaire for a survey, qualitative interviews would be used in the initial stages to identify salient issues for respondents and to develop questions that used the vocabulary of intended respondents.

One example is a large national survey of sexual behaviour in the UK conducted by Kaye Wellings and colleagues in part to provide essential information for planning health promotion activities and health services to reduce HIV infection (Wellings et al. 1994). The aims of the survey included quantifying aspects of individuals' sexual histories, measuring the prevalence and distribution of different patterns of sexual orientation, and measuring attitudes towards sexual behaviour. As a large amount of personal information was needed from respondents, a face-to-face interview survey was planned. The first phase was a qualitative one, including 40 in-depth interviews. These interviews were used to explore how much sexual information people were willing to disclose, what vocabulary people commonly used to discuss sexual behaviour, and how various terms were understood. The research team found a wide diversity of terms used to describe sexual experiences, and wide variation in how particular expressions (such as 'having sex') were understood. They also found that interviewees were uncomfortable with the use of vernacular terms in a research context, although these terms were used in private conversation. This is all essential information for designing a survey interview that is acceptable to respondents, and capable of generating reliable and valid data across the population.

Adapting existing survey instruments for new populations also requires qualitative research to improve the validity, reliability and sensitivity of the instrument. Annabel Bowden and colleagues (Bowden et al. 2002) discuss the challenges of developing a culturally sensitive measure of 'health' for use in studies evaluating the impact of interventions, in their case in Kenya. This kind of instrument would be largely used in quantitative studies, in order to measure the self-perceived health status of the target population following an intervention. However, as Bowden and colleagues argue, considerable qualitative research is needed to facilitate this. Many individual components of their study use qualitative methods to improve the survey instrument design. First, they drew on extensive anthropological participant observation studies to conceptualize 'health' from the perspective of the Kamba community in eastern Kenya. Second, they used interviews to aid in pre-testing potential questionnaire questions. In these, respondents were asked the survey question, and then prompted for their comprehension of key phrases and for their views on how appropriate the question was for respondents of different age and gender. Third, group interviews were used to generate discussion around some key issues in the survey. These allowed the researchers to access not just individual interpretations of questions, but also how opposing suggestions were debated. One such issue was what a 'family' comprised. The researchers used the local word for 'homestead', but found that even this had different meanings for different members, or even across different survey questions.

One contribution of qualitative methods to research programmes is, then, in the development phases, to provide data on feasibility, to generate hypotheses, or to do the developmental groundwork for new, or adapted, survey questionnaires.

Adding 'depth' or understanding findings from quantitative data

The second logical position a qualitative study can have within a broader programme is as a successor to quantitative work. Survey data might identify a relationship between variables, for instance, but may not be able to uncover the mechanisms – why they are linked. Case Study 2.1 is an example of qualitative research contributing in this way, to explore the reasons why women living on low incomes in the UK might smoke. Case Study 1.2 also used qualitative data to explore the meaning of quantitative data on outcomes. Similarly, qualitative research has had a vital role in understanding the 'meaning' of quantitative records, in terms of uncovering the processes by which the statistics that are used routinely in public health are produced. Data such as mortality rates, birth weight, population data and health service utilization statistics are often used routinely in health service planning, with only superficial consideration of the problems with reliability and validity. Qualitative work can identify the social factors that shape how these are both produced and used, providing some understanding of how valid they are.

Gillian Lewando-Hundt and colleagues (Lewando-Hundt et al. 1999; Lewando-Hundt 2001), for instance, used observational methods to examine the social context of birth registration in Gaza. Having intended to use information recorded on birth certificates for identifying a sample of mothers to interview, they found that the address listed on the certificate was always either incomplete or inaccurate, although the date and place of birth of babies was recorded correctly. Following the pathways information took to get recorded officially on a birth certificate, the researchers found that clerks actually used the father's registered address for the birth certificate, even if this was different from the baby's, as the birth certificate would be rejected by the Ministry of the Interior if the two addresses were different. Other social and political incentives for not recording addresses accurately also suggested that interventions to improve registration would be unlikely to work. There were, for instance, few street names or house numbers at that time in the Gaza Strip, as most had been removed during the *intifada* and the Palestinian population might be cautious about any records making them easier to locate. A second problem was recorded birth weights. These were often missing from hospital discharge sheets, as doctors reported being too busy to complete them, so some clerks would leave a blank on the form. Another, though, said he would fill in a nominal weight of 3 kg. This is essential information for epidemiological research, yet this study suggests likely systematic biases in its collection mean that low birth weight in Gaza is underestimated. This example demonstrates the value of qualitative methods as a way of unpacking the meaning of statistical records.

Parallel studies

Finally, qualitative and quantitative research questions on the same topic may be undertaken simultaneously, with the aim of extending our understanding of a phenomenon. Brent Wolff and colleagues (1993) argue that even though surveys and focus groups (see Chapter 5) are rooted in different theoretical approaches, they can be used as complementary methods within a single research study. They illustrate the benefits from their own study of the consequences of fertility in decline on families in Thailand. This study aimed to explore the relationship between family size and three outcomes: educational attainment of children, wealth accumulation, and the economic role of women. Wolff and colleagues discuss three ways in which the two elements added to the study. First, data from the focus groups illustrated survey findings, providing 'colour' to the statistical associations found in the quantitative data. Second, focus group findings helped clarify survey results. For example, one apparently contradictory finding from their survey was that although the majority of respondents felt that smaller families enjoy a relative economic advantage, a significant number also felt that if their family was larger, they would own more consumer goods. Focus groups enabled the researchers to see that position in the life course was critical to understanding the role of the number of children in wealth accumulation (whether they lived at home or were married and had left) and the role of children in persuading families to buy consumer goods. Third, focus groups raised new explanations that would not have arisen from the survey data. One example was the impact of child care on women's productivity in agricultural work. Even though variables such as number of children and length of time away from agricultural work for each could be quantified, the impact of child care on productivity could not, so the qualitative study provided this kind of detail. Here, qualitative and quantitative designs are used simultaneously to contribute different perspectives on the same problem.

Conclusion: developing skills in research design

Designing feasible, interesting and useful qualitative health research projects is probably the most difficult part of the whole research process, and one that is often inadequately done. In part, this is because it is difficult to develop clear guidelines for many of the important steps, such as refining the research question. Martin Bulmer, for instance, discusses the problem of describing how concepts in research questions are formed and refined. Noting that many of the concepts that social scientists use are complex and rich in meaning, he says:

> Concept-formation . . . proceeds neither from observation to category, nor from category to observation, but in both directions at once and in interaction. The distinctive character of concepts in empirical social science derives from this dual theoretical and empirical character. (Bulmer 1984: 44)

The work entailed in thinking about the concepts of interest (such as health behaviours, beliefs, health service utilization or communication) involves both reflecting on theory and on empirical evidence. This chapter has outlined some starting points for this process, in suggesting some questions that researchers can ask themselves when starting out on designing qualitative studies. A final suggestion is that working with others can be a productive way of developing your own design. Colleagues can suggest other theoretical and epistemological starting points and, in doing so, help test your assumptions. Explaining the logic of your design to them will help you clarify exactly what it is you are hoping to do. Once the research design has been adequately developed, you should be able to explain to a non–specialist what you want to find out, how you will do this, and why.

KEY POINTS

- A good research design is a coherent argument for how the data generated will answer a research question.
- Although many qualitative studies use flexible and less formal designs, in health research relatively formal protocols are usually required.
- Refining your research question involves reflecting on the concepts of interest and how you will generate data that reflects components of these (indicators).
- There are a number of dimensions along which research designs could be classified – we suggest a pragmatic typology based on aims of the study: experiments, surveys, observational studies, case studies and action research.
- There is no necessary relationship between the design and methods of data collection.

EXERCISES

1   From your own experiences of health care, either as a patient or a provider, identify some potential research topics, based on 'puzzles' you have about patient or provider behaviour.

2   Take one of these that relates to qualitative questions, and refine it as a research question. Consider the concepts of interest, what components of these concepts would be researchable, and how you would find evidence of them.

3   Design a small research project that would enable your research question to be answered. What factors do you need to take into account? What assumptions are underpinning your design? Which methods would be most suitable for collecting the data you think necessary?

FURTHER READING

Silverman, D. (2000) *Doing qualitative research: a practical handbook*. London: Sage. This draws on student diaries of their research experiences to look in a grounded way at the decisions that have to be made about design and choice of methods. Includes chapters on the research experience, selecting a topic and writing research proposals.

Patton, M.Q. (1990) *Qualitative evaluation and research methods* (2nd ed.). Newbury Park, CA: Sage. This is orientated more towards practical evaluation studies, but has a comprehensive chapter on research design covering various typologies of research and the choices between designs and data collection methods.

3

Responsibilities, Ethics and Values

CHAPTER SUMMARY

Ethical research practice requires a consideration of responsibilities to research participants, professional and academic colleagues, research sponsors and the wider public. Although ethical guidelines exist for most disciplines, qualitative health research often generates ethical dilemmas, which are not easily solved by reference to codes of practice. This chapter discusses the kinds of decisions qualitative health researchers have to make in designing studies that address their often conflicting responsibilities to different stakeholders.

Introduction

Any research study involves a number of different stakeholders, potentially including the research team and the institution for which they work, the professional organizations they may represent, the participants, the sponsor, policy-makers who may use results, various groups affected by those results, and the wider public, who pay for much health research. Meeting the diverse needs of these stakeholders generates a number of questions and (sometimes) conflicts about responsibilities and values. Who is the research ultimately for: the participants who helped generate the data, the wider community, knowledge for its own sake, or the research funder? How should it be conducted: is the researcher the expert, who should decide all aspects of methodology, or should participants have a role in shaping the research questions and data collection methods? How should findings be disseminated, and whose interests must be protected while doing this? What happens when our contractual obligations to sponsors (for instance not to publish until they have approved a report) conflict with our professional obligations to disseminate widely? What happens if we come across cases of poor clinical practice while doing fieldwork – do our professional obligations to protect patients override our responsibilities as researchers to protect the confidentiality of our informants? There are no clear 'rules' for deciding how to deal with these kinds of ethical dilemmas. However, researchers do have a duty perhaps to be informed about areas of ethical conflict, so that they can engage in open debate about the issues their research is likely to generate at the outset of the study. This chapter discusses the key issues of values, responsibilities and ethics raised by conducting qualitative research on health.

A first source of potential tension arises from different models of what research is *for* at a general level, which each imply some rather different ideas about the proper responsibilities of researchers.

Values in research

A positivist view of science is of investigative endeavour that somehow lies outside human values, and searches for an untainted 'truth' without reference to political or social influences. This is of course an ideal, as all science is rooted in social values. The topics that are held to be worthy of research, the kinds of questions that emerge as 'problems' to be addressed, the ways in which they can be legitimately researched, and the likelihood of publication of the findings are functions of the current social, political and cultural interests. However, the notion of the 'ivory tower' researcher who can pursue research questions to produce knowledge for its own sake, without the constraints of policy and politics, persists as one ideal to strive for, and as a pervasive influence on some approaches to research ethics. In this view, the responsibilities of the researcher are to conduct research in a scientifically sound way, and questions about what happens to the results are less important: the policy implications of findings are not the task of researchers, but of other social actors. To some extent, many disciplinary codes of ethics lean towards this model, and often focus on ensuring the scientific soundness of research, rather than considering its social implications. The statement of ethical practice of the British Sociological Association, for instance, although mostly dealing with responsibilities to participants, also contains several exhortations to members on professional integrity. Members, it says, should

> strive to maintain the integrity of sociological enquiry ... and to publish and promote the results of sociological research ... they should not accept work of a kind they are not qualified to carry out ... they should satisfy themselves that the research they undertake is worthwhile ... [they] should be careful not to claim an expertise in areas outside those that would be recognised academically as their true fields of expertise ... members should have regard for the reputation of their discipline. (BSA 1992)

As a 'scientist', then, of whatever discipline, the researcher has an obligation to 'do good science' and the primary responsibility is to 'knowledge' in an abstract sense, and perhaps to future generations of researchers. The implications this has for research practice are secondary. For instance, it would be important to carry out research in a way sensitive to the needs of participants in the field – but primarily so as not to 'spoil the pitch' for future researchers.

A weaker liberal approach holds that ethical values cannot be absolute, and that therefore ethical practice is relative and dependent on the moral professionalism of the researcher. Just as 'science' is not the value-free, objective system it is often claimed to be, so 'ethical principles' are not universals. In clinical medicine and public health, for example, ethical debate often takes the 'four principles' of Tom Beauchamp and Jim Childress (1983) as a starting point, which are rooted in health care ethics:

- autonomy – respecting the rights of the individual;
- beneficence – doing good;
- non-maleficence – not doing harm;
- justice – particularly distributive justice or equity.

These are, for most of us, laudable aims, but the language used to formulate them suggests they are somehow ancient and natural laws, rather than the constructions of a particular historical and cultural setting, such as Western liberal democracy (see, for instance, Gillon 1994 for some perspectives that differ from these as foundational principles). These principles arise from a consideration of medical practice and the individual patient, where it is perhaps relatively straightforward to balance potential good against potential harm, or to respect autonomy. They may be less useful as guides to decision-making in complex health research settings, when the 'good' for future patients may have to be measured against the autonomy of current participants, for instance. In the liberal view, decisions about what to research, how to do it and how to publish must be made at the discretion of the researcher, whose conscience should be the primary guide. Roger Homan (1991), in his book on social research ethics, advocates one version of this position: that social research needs to develop what he calls a 'professional morality' around 'quality control ... and a commitment to truth and knowledge' (1991: 183). For Homan, there will always be conflicts between the individual scruples of researchers (over, for instance, from whom they will accept funding, or what methods they think justified) and the public need to know. It would be impossible for ethical codes to legislate effectively for all eventualities and potential conflicts of interest, and in any case professional codes are likely to be in the interests of the profession, rather than the public. It would, then, be difficult to determine any normative ethical principles for social research, and we need instead, argues Homan, to develop a professional commitment to ethical practice built on an understanding of the dilemmas involved.

A third position is an overtly partisan one, believing that research should be carried out with the explicit aim of contributing to social justice, or emancipation. As Howard Becker put it, in a classic statement of the partisan position, 'The question is not whether we should take sides, since we inevitably will, but rather whose side are we on?' (Becker 1967: 239). His answer was that we should take the side of 'the underdog'. He argued that society is marked by what he called a 'hierarchy of credibility', which makes the views of those of higher status more 'credible' than those further down the social scale. The assumptions of a common-sense view of the world are that those at the top of any established order have a less biased view than those at the bottom. Thus the views of adults are believed over those of children, those of chief executives over the shop-floor workers, and those of medical professionals over patients. Therefore, argues Becker, the job of the social scientist is to query the established order, reveal the hierarchy of credibility for what it is and, in our research, give more credence to the views of the 'underdogs' to redress the bias that goes unremarked in most accounts of the social world.

Although perhaps attractive to some for its overtly political stance, there are considerable problems with Becker's position. First, there are of course multiple and complex hierarchies in most social settings. If we are to take the side of patients rather than their doctors, we must ask 'which patients?'. Annette Lawson (1991), for instance, in taking issue with Becker's account, discusses her experience of doing research for a voluntary organization representing those with multiple sclerosis. Although as patients these participants would be the 'underdogs' of Becker's hierarchy, the voluntary organization was in fact a well-funded and relatively powerful one, which meant they had considerable power over the research agenda. In addition, different patient groups had very different views on the research aims, so it was not possible to identify one homogeneous 'underdog' perspective. Lawson also notes the institutional changes that have happened over the decades since Becker's account was published, which have shifted the focus of research towards a more obviously policy-relevant agenda. Continued funding, and thus employment for researchers, relies on being seen as producing 'useful' and credible findings that are not obviously tied to the interests of one group or another.

In short, the debates around the proper responsibilities of researchers could be summarized as three broad positions that can be adopted as starting points for ethical decisions. These positions contain rather different assumptions about the relationship between research and society that is either possible or desirable. They are:

1   *The 'neutral outsider'*. Researchers should strive to be disinterested in political
     and social values, given that their role is to produce knowledge for its own
     sake. The implications of that knowledge, and the impacts it has on society, are
     not the proper concern of the researcher.
2   *The 'liberal relativist'*. As ethical standards are differently constructed across
     different settings, researchers should follow their own (professional) conscience
     in deciding what to research and how to do it.
3   *The 'radical'*. The proper role of research is to improve society, and the
     researcher should be explicitly partisan about their practice, striving to redress
     inequalities and increase social justice through their research practice. Of
     course, researchers can be partisan from conservative political positions as
     well, although more generally research from the position of the status quo is
     able to position itself as 'neutral'.

In practice, few researchers would locate themselves exclusively within one
of these positions, and the approach taken may well shift between different
projects. In reviewing these various positions on the proper role of researchers
in relation to social and political values, David Silverman (1985) criticizes all of
them for what he calls a 'self-righteousness' about the role of social research.
Instead, he suggests a more modest question around values that should be the
starting point. Rather than asking whether or not we should take sides, we
should, he suggests, ask what we can contribute. This is in many ways a neat
side-stepping of the issue, and certainly a more answerable question. As the
previous two chapters have suggested, the potential contributions of qualitative
research to our understanding of health and health care are diverse, and at a
number of different levels: the key issue about values becomes one of identifying the potential contribution, rather than positioning the research in terms of
political standpoints. However, the question of identifying potential contributions does not absolve the researcher from considering often difficult issues
around ethics and responsibilities that are raised by all research. The particular
'contribution' is of course usually tied to specific political or policy positions.
We still have to consider various sets of responsibilities, and are sometimes
faced with difficult decisions about the 'right thing to do'.

Deciding on the 'right thing to do' in research practice involves a consideration of the immediate impact on research participants and colleagues, longer-
term potential impacts on communities that could be affected, and responsibilities to both research sponsors and to professional and academic colleagues.
These various stakeholders in the research process might have rather different
interests, and the various models of ethical practice outlined above imply that
those of different stakeholders would be stressed. The 'neutral outsider' would
see the primary stakeholder as the discipline, and the primary responsibility of
the researcher is to contribute knowledge to that discipline. The 'liberal relativist's' primary responsibility is to their own conscience. That of the 'radical' is
to the participants and society more widely. If we follow Silverman, and
instead ask where our contribution lies, then we see our primary responsibility

to the users and funders of research. The various stakeholders have different, sometimes conflicting, interests in the research process, and one task of ethical reviews is to adjudicate between them: to balance society's need for knowledge against the rights of individuals involved in the research, or obligations to professional colleagues against the needs of sponsors.

Ethical review and codes of practice

What constitutes 'ethical practice' is different in different places and times, and across different disciplines. It is, then, impossible and perhaps even undesirable to develop a set of criteria that will ensure that a study is 'ethical' if they are met. Instead, there a number of issues raised by doing qualitative work that must be considered in the context of each particular study. First, this context will include a number of more or less formal frameworks that determine what kinds of research activity can and can't be done:

- *Legal frameworks.* National law may have an impact on issues such as confidentiality of data, and responsibilities to particular groups of participants, such as children.
- *Disciplinary codes of practice* governing research activity. The research activity of those in professions such as nursing and medicine is usually governed by professional codes of ethics. The professional associations of social scientists in many countries also issue ethical guidelines, which are usually advisory rather than mandatory.
- Local *cultural norms of ethical conduct* in both the fieldwork setting and the researcher's institution.
- Formal *ethical review*, through ethics committees.

In many institutional settings, ethical review is a formal process, requiring approval from an ethics committee before any study can start. This is part of research governance, in which institutions monitor standards of good practice and ensure that the relevant codes of practice are upheld. In the UK, for instance, the Department of Health issues guidance for local Research Ethics Committees, which are responsible for approving any study that involves users or staff of the National Health Service. Their role is primarily to consider the interests of research participants, but also to ensure that any proposed studies use appropriate designs for reaching sound conclusions (DOH 2001). Difficulties arise when there are conflicts between these various frameworks. Within the NHS, for instance, local Research Ethics Committees are primarily concerned with clinical research, and may have little experience in judging the appropriateness of qualitative designs. The local norms of the fieldwork setting may be very different from those of the institution, and the ethical guidelines of professional associations may not be in line with those of the institution's ethics committee.

In health research, many researchers are working within health care institutions or medical schools that are concerned primarily with the implications of medical research. Medical research is in general more tightly governed than other kinds of research, and guidelines developed for the conduct of research on medical subjects have a long history, starting from the Nuremberg Trials of 1947. This trial of the 23 doctors accused of atrocities committed during the Second World War resulted in the Nuremberg Code, which established principles of medical research including voluntary participation, informed consent and the justification of any risks expected (Homan 1991). Since then, issues of confidentiality and privacy have been added to most ethical codes. Internationally, for instance, the Declaration of Helsinki (WMA 2000) sets out ethical principles for medical research for the World Medical Association. This begins by placing the well-being of the 'human subject' above the interests of science and society. Researchers have a duty to protect the life, health, privacy and dignity of the human subject and to seek ethical review for all research protocols.

To carry out any work within health care settings may require the approval of an ethics committee, which will use criteria based on these principles taken from medical research guidelines. Social research in many countries has been less regulated, with fewer formal mechanisms to vet the ethics of proposed studies. As ethics committees are more familiar with medical research such as drug trials, the criteria they apply may work less well for qualitative social research on health. Even the language used may be rather inappropriate. Medical ethics committees, for instance, tend to refer to research 'subjects' rather than participants. The criteria may be very detailed on issues around potential biomedical risks, but less useful on the sorts of issues that are faced by ethnography, or using flexible research designs.

For social research, professional bodies such as the British Sociological Association (BSA 1992) and the Association of Social Anthropologists (ASA 1987) also have ethical guidelines, although in most countries these are more likely to be advisory and informative than mandatory. The ethical approval of social research is generally left to individual institutions rather than professional bodies.

Although medical and social research ethical guidelines have differing emphases, two key principles common to both, and included in most codes of ethics, are *informed consent* and *confidentiality*. Although both are perhaps uncontroversial as principles, they do generate some difficult decisions in practice with many qualitative designs.

Principle of informed consent

Informed consent is the principle that individuals should not be coerced, or persuaded, or induced, into research 'against their will', but that their participation should be based on voluntarism, and on a full understanding of the implications of participation. Homan (1991: 71) suggests that there are four components to the concept of 'informed consent'. 'Informed' implies both that all pertinent aspects of what will happen are disclosed to the participant, and that they are able to comprehend the information. 'Consent' implies that the participant is capable of making a rational judgement about whether to participate, and that their agreement should be voluntary rather than the result of coercion or undue influence.

Informed consent has been a cornerstone of most sets of ethical guidelines since the Nuremberg Code. The first of ten rules for the ethical conduct of medical experiments sets out the principle of voluntary and informed participation (Homan 1991), and these have been endorsed by medical professionals through the various revisions of the Declaration of Helsinki (WMA 2000), which states that 'subjects *must* be volunteers and informed participants' (point 20, emphasis added). Similar criteria are a basic principle of all professional guidelines for conducting research, such as the British Sociological Association (BSA 1992), which states: '*as far as possible*, sociological research should be based on freely given informed consent' (BSA 1992, emphasis added).

The 'as far as possible' reflects the broad range of research designs in social research, whereas the stricter criteria of Helsinki and other medical codes assume perhaps an intervention design, in which the 'research' activity is easily separated from other areas of social life. In a traditional experiment, such as a drug trial, it is relatively easy to inform participants of the aims of a study, which are fixed at the outset, and for the participants to know when they are being experimented on. In many qualitative designs, data will come from a range of informants, and it may be difficult to know at the time whether an opportunistic interview in the field will be 'data' in a formal sense. Further, some observational designs are based on observing people in public settings, where it would be very difficult to secure consent at the outset. Local sets of guidelines (such as those of institutional ethics committees) often attempt to operationalize what 'informed' should mean. This might include guidelines that list the kind of information that should generally be given to participants, including the objective of the study, who is funding and conducting it, the risks involved, how the data will be handled, and who can be contacted for further information.

Despite a high degree of consensus that informed consent is a worthwhile principle, there is considerable debate over what this means in practice. Given the complexity of research designs often used in health care research, how far do we go in informing research participants about the study aims? Research on how participants understand terms such as 'randomization' and 'trial' has suggested that these can be understood very differently from how the research team might use them (Snowdon et al. 1997). In ethnographic studies, where the aims may shift during the process of data collection and analysis, how far should researchers go in keeping their participants informed about changing emphases? Increasingly, ethics committees require researchers to provide written evidence of informed consent unless there are good reasons not to (such as a non-literate population). However, the very act of asking someone to sign a form can, in many cultures, undermine the research relationship, as illustrated in Case Study 3.1.

A further problem for many ethnographic or participatory designs is that participants may not be recruited to a study as individuals, but as collectivities, such as staff on a hospital ward, or members of a patients' organization. Here, gaining informed consent can pose practical difficulties, in that the participants change over the period of fieldwork, and new people enter the field at various points. Carrying out participant observation on a ward, for example, may involve not only informing nursing, medical, clerical and cleaning staff but also those who may come onto the ward occasionally, such as physiotherapists or porters, and locum or agency staff, as well as patients and their visitors. Although regular meetings at shift hand-overs can be a useful way to re-negotiate consent throughout the fieldwork period, it can be very difficult to make sure everyone contributing to the emerging data set is truly informed about the study.

Multiple gatekeepers present similar problems in situations where direct access to study participants is not possible. Gatekeepers are those who control the researcher's access to the fieldwork site or to other participants, either formally, in cases such as managers whose support will be needed to gain access to a hospital, or informally to aid recruitment of hard to reach groups, or to legitimize the study. Examples might include community leaders who can help inform their communities about your study, or employers who can help recruit their employees. Although such gatekeepers are an essential route for gaining entry to many settings, they are of course also influential on the final partici-pants, and indeed are often chosen for their persuasiveness or support for the research. Individual participants may find it difficult to refuse to take part if an influential community leader or their employer has encouraged participation. Research with young people in schools is a good example. Here, permission might be needed from a hierarchy of gatekeepers, such as the local authority responsible for schools in the area, head teachers, class teachers, parents, and only finally the children. Although consent from the participating individual should be secured, it may be very difficult for young people to refuse to participate if their teachers and parents have given their permission. If one potential danger of the use of gatekeepers is that of undue pressure to partici-pate, the other (less commonly considered) is the opposite: that use of gate-keepers can restrict who is invited to take part. In the school setting, for instance, there may be a requirement to have parental consent before children are approached, meaning some young people who may want to participate may not even be given the opportunity to consider it.

The use of gatekeepers to aid and legitimate access is a necessity in many studies, but the researchers should strive both to ensure that participants are truly voluntary, and that the voices of particular individuals or groups are not being silenced by dependence on gatekeepers for contacts.

Confidentiality

The Helsinki Declaration notes that 'Every precaution should be taken to respect the privacy of the subject [and] the confidentiality of the patient's information' (WMA 2000). Social research ethics also stress confidentiality as a key criterion for ethical practice.

This first means not disclosing information gained from research in other settings, such as informal conversation. Some research designs make this more difficult than others. In participatory designs, for instance, it may be difficult to separate out information provided by participants as 'confidential' research information from routine information that is to be shared. Doing research close to home also makes confidentiality a difficult issue. Many researchers choose research questions arising from their personal or professional lives, and initial ideas for a project come from everyday conversations with collea-gues or friends. Clearly the ordinary social rules of confidentiality will apply to information given in this way, but once an area of interest has become a 'research study', there are perhaps additional obligations. If pilot interviews are carried out with colleagues or acquaintances, it is particularly important not to let information given here slip into everyday gossip.

Second, confidentiality relates to published accounts of the research, in which the identity of the sites and individuals should be protected where possible. Names and other identifiers can be changed to protect the privacy of participants. Case studies and evaluations of innovative service provisions present particular challenges in terms of anonymity. In straightforward evalua-tive studies, the site may well be named and consent will have been secured on the understanding that the final report will be of that site. In many settings, this means that individuals may be identifiable as well — there may only be one manager, or one health visitor, so qualitative accounts using quotes must be done very carefully, with the consent of those quoted. Research based on a single case, especially if an atypical one, is more problematic. To preserve enough detail to give the reader sufficient context to understand the findings may mean that anonymity, and therefore confidentiality, is difficult to main-tain. Ideally, such issues need to be discussed fully with participants at the outset, so that any assurances of anonymity and confidentiality are realistic, or the researcher may find publication impossible. Some participants may not want confidentiality. Anne Grinyer (2002), for instance, reports how in her research with parents of young people with cancer, many participants actively requested the use of their own and their children's real names. Otherwise, they felt, they lost ownership of a deeply personal story.

Another constraint on confidentiality comes from legal frameworks. It is difficult to give absolute guarantees of confidentiality, as there are situations in which there may be an obligation (moral if not legal) to break this. One example might be research with children, to whom the researcher has a responsibility as an adult, as well as a researcher. If a child being interviewed were to indicate that they were at risk in some way (for instance from parental abuse), many ethicists would see the primary duty of the researcher as one of safeguarding the child's safety, rather than their privacy. In some countries this would be a legal responsibility. If this is the case, researchers cannot offer complete confidentiality to young people in research settings. In settings where the researcher has no legal obligation to breach confidentiality, there is a difficult judgement call involving the degree of likely risk. For research with vulnerable groups such as children, it is good practice to establish protocols for these events at the beginning of a study, with a nominated person for the interviewers or research staff to contact in the first instance with concerns.

For some professionals, the discovery of very poor practice while doing fieldwork would constitute a similar dilemma in terms of whether to break confidentiality. If patients are being abused, or professionals are incompetent, should the researcher disclose this information? The answer to this may depend on a fine judgement of the likely risks to individuals in the research setting and the likely benefits arising from the research findings. Confidentiality should not be breached lightly: future participation relies on a climate of trust, and the researcher is not an auditor of good practice (unless this is the aim of the study).

Responsibilities to research participants

Consent and confidentiality are core principles that inform the responsibilities of researchers to the participants in research, but they are not the only issues to consider. Although social research is unlikely to generate risks to physical health, there are other, less obvious, impacts that need to be thought through, especially if the research is on a sensitive topic. This section considers the particular responsibilities to research participants raised in interview and ethnographic studies.

Ethics in interviews

The primary responsibility enshrined in most codes of ethics is to participants in the research: those who are interviewed, observed or who have contributed time and effort to the study. Although most qualitative research does not involve interventions that appear to impact directly on the lives of participants, we should not forget that involvement in research can have emotional consequences, particularly if the research concerns experiences of ill health, traumatic incidents, or issues normally considered 'private', such as sexual behaviour.

If qualitative research is built on respect for participants' world-views, data collection methods do have to convey this respect. This might involve, for instance, making sure interview questions reflect the concerns of interviewees, rather than merely pursuing the researcher's perspective. Kathryn Ehrich, a sociologist who reports on her experience of being on the receiving end of being interviewed, notes the discomfort she and her partner experienced as interviewees when an interviewer pursued a research agenda on the impact of chronic illness on families, without acknowledging the experiences that were most salient to them as 'respondents':

> ... we found that the research agenda was fully theirs, with no space for asserting our own experience of living with chronic illness. There was no dialogue, only the opportunity to answer questions co-operatively or not. My response was increasingly the latter, and I felt misunderstood, as though they thought I was presenting 'resistance'. ... Our focus was simply not of particular interest. (Ehrich 2001: 23)

When interviewing is done with regard to the interviewees' agenda, with empathy and understanding, it can be a very positive experience for participants, with many people pleased that someone is taking an interest in their lives and concerns. In her study of the transition to motherhood, for instance, Ann Oakley (1981) reported that the majority of her interviewees felt that the interviews had been a good experience, giving them an opportunity to talk about concerns and to reflect on their experiences. One exception may be members of particular groups who may become 'over-researched', and asked to take part in multiple studies. This can be particularly distressing if researchers raise expectations of, say, service improvements that are never realized.

One ethical problem in interview studies is that the tenets of 'good' interviewing practice (see Chapter 4) are those of encouraging trust and disclosure, the very skills that may make it most difficult for respondents to refuse, or to withdraw, once the interview has started. Good interviewers build a sense of rapport, and encourage interviewees to tell personal and detailed stories about themselves. They are, in short, experts at exploiting and mining individuals for data. For this to be done ethically, it has to be done with respect for the interviewee as an individual, rather than merely a carrier of 'good data'. The expert interviewer also has to remember to provide real opportunities to refuse, at any point. High response rates are often seen as an indicator of good-quality research, yet could just as easily be seen as evidence of inadequate possibilities for refusal or withdrawal. The researcher may have to balance the 'scientific' needs of a representative sample with the ethical needs to ensure proper consent is given, on an ongoing basis, to participation. They may also have to balance the scientific need for 'good data' against the possible risks to the participants of disclosure. Case Study 3.1, from rural India, is an example of a setting in which the research team had to be particularly careful of 'over-disclosure' on the part of their interviewees, in this case in focus group interviews.

Particular care should be taken when interviewing participants who are in a relatively powerless position compared with the researcher or those whose cognitive abilities are impaired. The latter may be less able to be 'informed' while the former may be less able to positively 'consent' to participation. Both situations may require imaginative steps to maximize true voluntary consent, but they do not preclude research with groups such as those with mental

Case Study 3.1   Cultural sensitivity and ethical practice: an example from rural India

(Source: Vissandjée, B., Abdool, S. and Dupéré, S. (2002) 'Focus groups in rural Gujarat, India: a modified approach', *Qualitative Health Research*, 12: 826–43)

Bilkis Vissandjée, Shelley Abdool and Sophie Dupéré discuss the appropriateness of focus groups (see Chapter 5) for their research on women's autonomy and health behaviour in rural India, in part because of strong local oral traditions. However, they also note that the method must be adapted for local conditions, taking into account the research topic, participants, and the social, political and cultural context of the study area. This raises a number of ethical considerations for researchers, who must think through how to adapt research designs in order to facilitate relatively disempowered participants in expressing their views, and ensuring that the research is conducted in an appropriate ethical manner – that it is 'culturally competent'.

   The project setting for their study was a rural area of Gujarat, with 25 relatively small villages that had little contact with outsiders. The research team were aware that this posed potential problems in establishing good relationships. First, villagers might be distrustful of outsiders, especially those from outside the country (there were Canadian researchers on the team) who might hold negative views of Indian society. Second, the topics they were asking women to discuss were not traditionally those on which women were encouraged to hold views, and some local men were concerned that the researchers were intending to 'change' women. Finally, the presence of an overseas research team may raise (false) expectations of aid or policy action. To address these concerns, the researchers embarked on a period of field preparation, in which they built relationships with community leaders and members. They did this in partnership with a local Community Health Volunteer (CHV), who knew the local villagers well. The team were careful to match genders at this point, as it would not have been appropriate to have women walking unaccompanied through the villages, or for a male researcher to talk to the local women. The CHV also helped with focus group recruitment, aiding door-to-door recruitment of potential participants. Recruiting door to door was essential in rural areas; not only did it facilitate communication in an area with no telephones and limited literacy, but it enabled the researchers to ask women to participate in the presence of the men in the household, who might otherwise feel hostile about the groups.

   The researchers had to take into account local power relationships, including those of caste and family relationship. It was not culturally possible to hold separate group discussions for the different castes in the village, but in the groups higher-caste women inhibited lower-caste women from speaking. Similarly, mothers-in-law had more authority than daughters-in-law in discussions. Here, the composition of groups entails ethical decisions that offset the needs for cultural appropriateness (including everyone) with the needs for hearing disempowered voices. Vissandjée and colleagues note that even if they had run more homogeneous groups that included only low-status women, in an area where 'everybody knows everybody', women may feel that anything they say will be reported back, and still feel constrained in discussing their views.

Written consent to participation was inappropriate, so the research team gave only verbal assurances of confidentiality. Written papers, in this context, would be negatively associated with government documents.

The closeness of rural communities also has an impact on the researchers' ability to ensure confidentiality. The team had to consider how far they were responsible for any consequences of women's behaviour in the focus group, given that they would be seen as representatives of their families, and any disapproved behaviour or talk would probably be communicated back to the family. In these circumstances, the focus group moderator has to stress that the research team will treat the data generated with confidence, but also has to guard against 'over-disclosure' (participants feeling so comfortable that they reveal more than they had intended) in the group, given the possible future consequences for participating women. Given that the researchers were asking women to reflect on their own lives in ways that were potentially very destabilizing, it was also useful to provide follow-up opportunities for private discussion and reflection on participation in the group discussion.

Vissandjée and colleagues were working within a participatory approach, where the key ethical dilemmas faced were the need to balance 'empowerment' for women in the community with the potential risks to individual women as a result of their involvement in the project. One ethical risk of this kind of project, they note, is that once the researchers disappear, individual women may be left with a sense of developing awareness but with a dissatisfaction that there is nothing they can do, as they are too busy or isolated to discuss the issues raised with other women. An essential step to minimize the risk of this happening is to disseminate findings from the study at village level, and to work with local health care providers to develop follow-up local activities.

disabilities, limited language skills or powerless social positions. Indeed, one might argue that researchers have a duty to reflect the voices of those who are least likely to have other access to the public arena. Information about the project needs to be provided in ways appropriate for the participants, and this may mean using video or photographs rather than written forms.

To offset the power imbalance between researcher and interviewee, the interview format may need to be thought about carefully. First, the location is important. Given that most interviewees will feel relatively more empowered in their own environment than yours (Green and Hart 1999), the interviewee's home or other familiar place may be more suitable than a university office or clinic room. This is, of course, context specific: in some settings the home may be too crowded or lacking in privacy for one-to-one interviews. Case Study 5.1, which describes a study of Bedouin views of maternal health services, is a good example here, as Susan Beckerleg and her colleagues describe the inappropriateness of trying to do a 'private' interview in the home setting. Here, an institutional setting might be preferable if the topic were one that required privacy.

A second consideration in thinking about power in the research process is the interview format. A one-to-one interview can be intimidating, and interviewing people in pairs or small groups may redress the power imbalance. This is particularly useful when working with young people, who can be asked if they would like to do the interview with a friend or sibling. However, it is worth remembering that few interviewees are entirely powerless. In practice, most participants will have a number of strategies at their disposal for declining to participate without actually having to refuse. Adolescents, for instance, may be monosyllabic in answering questions, or rural villagers may deliberately divulge only misleading stories. Baker and Hinton quote one of the participants in their research, who was resentful of the many interviews she had previously been asked to take part in. Rather than refusing, she said her approach was to 'give a quick answer to let them go away' (Baker and Hinton 1999: 88).

Ethics in observational studies

Participant observation (see Chapter 6) involves the researcher participating to some extent in a social field (a village community, a hospital ward) in order to research it. The first ethical issue raised by using these methods in health care projects governed by medical ethics is that informed consent is often problematic. In a bounded field (such as one small clinic) it may be possible to secure consent from all parties. Most health care settings, however, involve changing staff and patients, and it is very difficult to ensure that all parties present at every point in the fieldwork are fully informed about the study and actively consenting to be research participants. Julienne Meyer (1993) discusses the limitations of informed consent in her action research study of lay participation in care in a London hospital ward. Finding a ward that would be willing to work with her for a year of fieldwork was a long task, but even with this careful preparation, Meyer has some reservations about consent. Once the project was underway, she notes, it would have been very difficult for an individual to withdraw as they are part of a group who made a commitment to work together. If a few individuals become uncomfortable with a project, would it be ethical to call a halt, given the input and commitment of the rest of the team?

Joan Cassell (1980) discusses the wide range of models adopted by anthropologists doing fieldwork, and suggests that the key principle for informing ethical practice should be respect for human autonomy. Medical research ethics primarily entail assessing the risks for harm to 'subjects', but this, she argues, is an inappropriate rubric for anthropologists. First, assessing the likely 'harm' is very difficult, and second, the kind of 'harm' caused by social research usually relates to hurt feelings, or invasions of privacy, rather than the kinds of injury or physical harm resulting from medical interventions. Although anthropologists should of course take all steps possible to remove the risk of harm, the more important principle should be the attempt to treat people as autonomous agents, rather than means to ends. Thus, research practice that involves coercing people to participate in an interview, or deceiving them, would be difficult to justify ethically even if confidentiality was respected and there was no harm to the participant. A focus on respecting autonomy would make most covert studies questionable.

Covert methods

Covert methods, in which the researcher does not disclose their role to those in the field, clearly raises a number of particular ethical dilemmas. Not only is the autonomy of the participants not respected, but informed consent is impossible to secure, at least before the fieldwork. The use of covert methods is discussed in Chapter 6. One classic example is Rosenhan's (1973) study of psychiatric hospitals in the USA, which relied on research assistants gaining admission as patients by pretending to have symptoms, described in Case Study 3.2.

Rosenhan's study of psychiatric hospitals raises some interesting ethical issues. It clearly violates the principle of informed consent, and it is unlikely that many ethics committees today would approve such a study. However, the findings from his study could probably not have been gained in any other way. Although it could be argued that there are many detailed 'insider' accounts from 'real' hospital patients, both autobiographical and literary, these come from those stigmatized by the diagnosis of 'mental illness' and thus have less legitimacy than accounts from an academic team of researchers. Does this justify the deceit involved? One justification is the 'public interest' argument. Rosenhan's study may have had little immediate policy impact, but was part of the backdrop of cultural knowledge that influenced policies in many countries away from long-term hospitalization as a way of managing mental illness and towards community care. However, a real cost is the loss of trust between professionals and researchers.

Another argument that has been made in defence of these covert methods is that of cultural relativity: that ideas such as autonomy and privacy are tied to Western notions of individuality, and may be inappropriate in different settings. Justifying their covert study of a hospital ward in Ghana, van der Geest and Sarkodie (1998) argue that the very notion of 'informed consent' is a culture-bound one, and that in the Ghanaian context, especially in a rural environment, there is less concern with the notion of privacy. Although we would agree that notions of 'privacy' are of course culturally specific, and good research practice should involve identifying how they are locally constructed (as in Case Study 3.1), there are real ethical problems with applying different *standards* in different settings. In their paper, van der Geest and Sarkodie suggest that their practice (although not in line with anthropological codes of ethical

Case Study 3.2   Covert observation of psychiatric hospitals

(Source: Rosenhan, D.L. (1973) 'On being sane in insane places', *Science*, 179: 250–8)

Rosenhan was interested in how reliable and valid diagnostic measures of 'sanity' were, and whether psychiatric staff were able to distinguish the sane from the insane. He devised an experiment in which eight 'normal' people got themselves admitted to US psychiatric hospitals by claiming to hear voices that said 'hollow', 'empty' or 'thud', but by otherwise presenting their 'real' medical and social histories to admission clinic staff. All were admitted with a diagnosis of schizophrenia, except one with a diagnosis of manic depressive psychosis. On admission, the researchers behaved normally and co-operated with hospital routines. Given that they spent considerable time in the hospitals waiting to be discharged, their undercover status provided an opportunity for covert observation. Rosenhan's paper reports on their experiences of being hospitalized, and the ways in which the diagnostic label they had received at admission shaped the interpretation of their behaviour by staff. None of the researchers were identified as sane pseudo-patients by staff, although interestingly many other patients challenged them, assuming that they were undercover journalists or researchers. In general, they were discharged with diagnoses of 'schizophrenia in remission'.

Rosenhan's findings were important. Not only did he contribute to the debate around the social construction of labels such as schizophrenia, but the reports of his pseudo-patients were an important contribution to our understanding of the effects of both hospitalization and labelling. Labelling someone as mentally ill shapes the interpretation of all their behaviour. As patients with a diagnosis, the everyday behaviours of the researchers, such as writing notes or being anxious in the new hospital environment, were seen as symptoms of their disease. Rosenhan's descriptions of many aspects of hospitalization, such as the low level of interaction between staff and patients, the occasional abuse of patients and lack of privacy, were a significant development in our understanding of how institutions lead to depersonalization and may contribute to mental ill health, rather than cure it. With other studies of long-term institutions, this pseudo-patient study was an influence in the gradual policy shift in many countries away from asylums and towards other forms of care for those with mental health problems.

However, the design of the study raises a number of ethical questions. First, there are the problems of deceit. Except in one case, neither the hospital staff nor other patients knew that they were participants in the research (though some patients did guess), and had not consented to take part. Rosenhan defends the concealment (though he does admit it is 'distasteful') on the basis that it was necessary. It was the only way that these data could have been gathered. If hospitals were warned that researchers would try to get themselves admitted, there would be no way of knowing whether the process of admission and experiences on the wards were typical or not. The hospitals and staff are not named in the report: Rosenhan is not interested in exposing poor practice (as an undercover journalist might) but rather in generalizing from his data to say something about the ways in which mental illness is dealt with in the American health care system. The defence against breaching normal expectations of informed participation is thus a public interest one, based on utilitarian principles. In short, the ends (furthering public knowledge with the aim of improving services for some of the most marginalized people in society) could be argued to justify the means. Arguably, though, Rosenhan's study 'spoils the pitch' for future researchers attempting to study psychiatric services in more open ways, making mental health professionals defensive and less willing to consider change. If these disadvantages are taken into account, the benefit in terms of service improvements may be less likely. A final ethical consideration is the safety of the research team. Once admitted to the hospitals, most of the researchers wanted to leave very quickly, as they were unpleasant places to be. It is, however, difficult to get discharged at short notice, and they spent between 7 and 52 days as patients. This experience may be distressing, and there was also the danger of having to take unnecessary medications.

conduct) is justifiable because the research may lead to better hospital conditions for patients in Ghana. In other words, the ends justify the means. In terms of Cassell's focus on respect and autonomy discussed above, this would not of course be justifiable.

In terms of fieldwork practice, one source of debate over ethical positions is, then, between those who view the *process* as the key issue, and develop methodological strategies that maximize respect for human autonomy, and those who consider the *ends* to be the deciding factor. For the latter, decisions about ethics are made in a more utilitarian way, in terms of assessing the likely benefit to the people involved (such as improved services) or the wider community against the risks.

Anthropological research and representing the 'other'

The ethical issues of participant observation studies do not end with fieldwork. Responsibilities to participants continue in the writing up and dissemination of accounts, and researchers should consider carefully the likely impact not only on individual participants, but the likely policy impact of the study more broadly. This includes obvious considerations of confidentiality and being careful to disguise distinguishing characteristics. Circulating a draft report to informants can help identify any areas they feel may leave them vulnerable if identified.

Beyond the immediate concerns of embarrassment for individuals who may be identified in research reports, there are broader issues around representing communities. Nancy Scheper-Hughes (2000) gives a moving account of her attempts to write 'honest ethnography' whilst maintaining a respect for those she lived with for nearly a year. Returning to the Irish village community she studied twenty-five years previously, she is struck by how betrayed villagers still feel by the book she wrote of her experiences. The book, *Saints, Scholars and Schizophrenics*, was an exploration of how particular social structures and family patterns could be functional for society, but dysfunctional for individuals, making some vulnerable to mental ill health. Like any ethnography, it was, she notes, a partial view – as much reflecting her political and theoretical concerns as the views of the villagers. Reacting against a 'functionalist' tradition in anthropology, which stressed only the positive and functional aspects of culture, she brought a feminist and theoretically eclectic approach to exploring the dysfunctional aspects of rural community life against a historical backdrop of British colonialism, famine and the decline of agricultural economies. Despite attempts to disguise the identity of the community in her ethnography, it was identified by a journalist, and became visited by a number of other researchers in the intervening years. Reflecting on the controversy over the book, and the anger of villagers years later at what they saw as an overly negative portrayal that said nothing about the positive aspects of rural Irish culture, Scheper-Hughes suggests some of her ethical decisions would be different now. First, she would avoid pseudonyms and anonymity. These protect the anthropologist more than the participants, she argues, and perhaps mean we think less carefully about what we write. Second, there are the positive aspects of village life that could have been addressed as well – the absence of violence, close and enduring friendships, and social equality between men and women. Scheper-Hughes' experience illustrates the balancing act that many researchers face in meeting obligations to both communities (in representing them faithfully and not betraying close working relationships that have been built up over time) and the discipline (in analysing culture in ways that move forward our thinking about, say, the cultural roots of mental illness).

Different models of relationship

Participatory designs are built on the assumption that researching with, rather than on, people can change the power relationships inherent in the research enterprise, such that a more democratic relationship is established. Action research, as discussed in Chapter 2, is one potential participatory approach, given that the problem and solutions are identified not by an outside researcher, but by those in the field, with the researcher acting as facilitator rather than 'expert'. Julienne Meyer (1993) questions whether, in practice, this approach is in fact more democratic. In some ways it can lead to greater exploitation than traditional researcher–subject models, as the relationships between those in the field and the researcher are likely to be closer and more collaborative, therefore putting the participant in a potentially more vulnerable position. Further, the very experience of taking part in research, and having an outsider encourage questioning and reflection, might make for uncomfortable group dynamics as people reassess not only their own roles but those of others in the organization.

When a significant power imbalance between the researcher and the research participants generates ethical challenges for research, then participatory designs may be a useful way of finding a more responsible way of conducting the research. Virginia Morrow and Martin Richards (1996), for instance, suggest that participatory methods may be a good way of working with children. This might involve training young people themselves as interviewers so they can help shape the process of data collection with their peers and including young people's representatives on steering committees. Rachel Baker describes working with a 15-year-old former street child when researching the health and lives of street children in Nepal (Baker and Hinton 1999). This young man was in a position to talk with street children in a more equal way than the Western researchers, or workers from local agencies, although of course he was not an 'insider' in an unproblematic way. As the study described in Case Study 3.1 suggests, though, a participatory design does not solve the difficult issues of power imbalance within the community. In a rural Indian setting, Vissandjée and colleagues were interested in women's empowerment, and designed a participatory study to involve local villagers at all stages in the process. However, they had to work within both patriarchal and caste relationships in order to facilitate the research, and take account of power relationships within families. Further, they had no way of ensuring that by 'empowering' women in making them conscious of their own positions they were helping to dismantle any of those power dynamics. In short, participatory designs have to be thought through very carefully to ensure that researchers do not just compound social inequalities. Research is a very different enterprise from community development, and researchers should be wary of making extravagant claims about 'improving' communities unless they are really prepared to work long term in particular settings, rather than just carrying out one-off studies.

With rather less lofty aims, it is becoming more common to include the participants (or the wider community from whom they are selected) as recognized stakeholders in the research process, even if the design is not a participatory one. In the UK, researchers are often asked to include users or community representatives on steering groups for the project, or to build collaborative links with likely end users of the research, such as patient groups or local communities. The Association of Social Anthropologists (ASA 1987) has the involvement, as far as possible, of those being studied in both the design and conduct of the research as an ethical principle. There is, then, a principle of 'involving' users, as a 'good thing' in itself, even if not making claims about the virtue of this in terms of empowering research participants.

Responsibilities to yourself and co-workers

We have considered how responsibilities to participants have to be balanced against those of the public's 'right to know' and the potential future benefits to others. One set of responsibilities that are less often considered are those researchers have to themselves and co-workers at a personal as well as a professional level. At its most basic, there is a responsibility of personal safety. Traditionally, social researchers have often been rather cavalier about risks, and many of those working in the health field are working with agencies that operate in what could be seen as inherently risky environments, such as post-conflict settings or areas with epidemic disease. Increasingly, though, the health and safety of researchers as employees or students is being taken seriously by institutions, many of which will require a risk assessment to be carried out prior to fieldwork. If the sponsor or employing institution does not require risk assessment as a formal process, it is worth working through some of the potential risks faced with other members of the team and supervisors, particularly if you are planning on fieldwork in an unfamiliar setting. In a review of safety in research, Gary Craig, Anne Corden and Patricia Thornton (2000) suggest that researchers and those responsible for them think about the following sets of potential risks:

- Physical threats or abuse.
- Psychological trauma, including that arising from real or threatened violence or from what is disclosed during fieldwork.
- The potential for compromising situations, in which accusations of improper behaviour might be made.
- Increased exposure to risks such as infectious disease or accidental injury.

The aim of carrying out a risk assessment exercise is to identify and minimize the risks potentially faced by the research team, and to develop procedures for dealing with emergencies. The details will of course depend on the specific study: on the fieldwork environment, the data collection strategy and the support available in the study site. The risks faced by an ethnographer in a remote area of an unfamiliar country are rather different from those faced by an interviewer conducting research with managers in their own institution. Those planning projects in unfamiliar environments should consult widely with others who do know the setting. However, familiarity should not lead to complacency, as we are often less aware of risks on our home territory than we are in less familiar settings. Some common ways of minimizing the risks listed above might include:

- *Training.* Do fieldworkers need training in interpersonal skills needed to avoid conflict, cultural norms of the fieldwork site, or in any particular areas of risk assessment to do their job safely?

- *Maintaining contact with field staff.* Interviewers can leave itineraries with office staff or nominated individuals, and ensure that visits to interview sites are notified. The provision of mobile phones or phone cards may be worth considering, and regular e-mail contact with those based away from the host institution is advisable.
- *Debriefing.* Returning from a period of fieldwork can be emotionally difficult, and some form of debriefing should be organized. Equally, interviewing on sensitive or emotional topics can be traumatic, and some kind of support is needed, whether from colleagues or the supervisor.
- *Travel advice.* Adequate advice on travel health for those doing fieldwork away from home might include provision of health insurance, advice on immunizations needed and specialist advice on supplies such as mosquito nets or medicines.

Some of these considerations of personal safety have resource implications, and should be costed in at the outset of a study.

Ethical dilemmas and conflicts

So far, we have outlined various sets of responsibilities that researchers have, and a number of principles on which ethical decisions can be taken. We have suggested that ethical principles are not absolute, but are shaped by wider cultural values such that they vary across time and place. Privacy, for instance, was not addressed by early codes of ethical practice in medical research, but is now a core component in many professional codes, reflecting general social concern about data on individuals and how it is managed. Further, the practicalities of putting even widely agreed principles (such as consent) into practice have to be adapted to local norms, as shown in Case Study 3.1. The socially determined nature of ethical values means that it is not unusual for conflicts to arise over the proper way to manage a project, or to disseminate findings, with different stakeholders stressing different principles or disagreeing about how they should be enacted. In qualitative research on health, a first source of tension can be the different cultures of social and health research.

Social research and biomedical ethical practice

Much qualitative health research is done in multi-disciplinary teams, or across a number of institutions or countries, and these situations increase the chance that ethical dilemmas will arise about the 'right' thing to do. This chapter began with reference to codes of practice for medical and for social research. Although these codes of practice address the same issues, there may be differences across professions and research communities in what counts as ethical practice. One example is that of informed consent for young people. In medical research in the UK for people under 16 the consent of parents is required, but many community organizations working with young people would see this as undermining their autonomy. Qualitative research designs themselves often generate difficulties for ethics committees that have been set up to review biomedical research, in part because their flexibility and open-endedness can appear to be poor design, which would be difficult to justify in terms of the likely benefits to the participants. Biomedical ethics committees often consider research in terms of risks and benefits, rather than respect for the participants' autonomy. Even though the risks of social research may be low, the benefits can be hard to judge in instrumental ways.

The differences between the expectations of medical research and social science research communities also present potential dilemmas around data archiving. In many senses, archiving data for future researchers to use is good ethical practice: it is an efficient use of resources, avoids duplication of research effort, and leaves the study data potentially available for other analysts to look at, so increasing the generalizability of findings. In the UK, the Economic and Social Research Council (the main funders of social science research) encourages all researchers to archive in a national archive any qualitative data arising from their studies. However, many medical ethics committees will expect data to be destroyed at the end of a project to ensure confidentiality. Gill Backhouse (2002) advises researchers to deal with this dilemma by making sure data (such as transcripts) are anonymized, with identifying material removed, before they are prepared for archiving. She also encourages researchers to secure written consent from participants for archiving, and for participants to see transcripts for approval. Of course, in many research settings this will be difficult or inappropriate.

Whose risks?

Risk assessments are another potential source of ethical debate. Precautions that minimize risk for the researcher may in themselves recreate social prejudices about 'risky environments' – environments that are the homes and communities of those we are studying. What seem like sensible precautions for the researcher when interviewing in, say, a deprived inner-city estate (such as making contact with someone outside by mobile phone when entering or leaving, only interviewing during the daytime, or interviewing in pairs) may well feel like disrespect and suspicion to the resident of that estate. In addition, there is often a trade-off between 'safer' and 'more productive' data collection strategies. In participant observation studies in particular, the informal and opportunistic interviews and observations are often most useful, but of course these are the ones that might be avoided to maximize personal safety. Interviewing people in their own homes may be less safe than inviting them into the university, but may mean there is more chance of developing a trusting relationship.

Research in developing countries

We have already touched on the problem of dealing with local cultural norms when researching across different countries, and suggested that a distinction must be made between exploiting such differences (in, say, carrying out studies that would not be approved in the researcher's own country) and respecting differences (in designing culturally appropriate protocols). The Nuffield Council on Bioethics (NCB) (2003) looked at the issue of health care research in developing countries, and highlighted a number of potential risks of being 'sensitive to the local social and cultural context, while [needing] to ensure that their clinical methods reflect the obligations imposed by relevant national and international guidance' (NCB 2003: 134). The key issue, they suggested, is respect for difference, rather than necessarily adopting local practices if these would be considered unethical in most settings. One example might be that of senior members of a household consenting for, say, adult women. Sensitivity to local practice might suggest that heads of households are approached first, but ethical practice would require each individual's informed consent in addition. Although their report focused on the issues raised in clinical research, the general conclusions reached are perhaps applicable also to qualitative designs. They suggest four principles that should inform ethical practice: the duty to alleviate suffering, the duty to show respect for persons, the duty to be sensitive to cultural difference, and the duty not to exploit the vulnerable. Externally funded research in developing countries should, concludes the report, be ethically reviewed by a committee within the developing country which can ensure that the proposal fits with the health care priorities for that country, is scientifically valid and is ethically acceptable.

Commissioners and researchers

The different stakeholders in the research process may well have very different agendas, which may generate tensions for the researcher. Those who carry out and those who fund and commission research may be working with rather different models of what the research is for. Research for health is often commissioned by organizations that need timely findings disseminated as quickly as possible to address policy-relevant problems. However, researchers in academic settings may gain more credibility from generalizable, theoretically driven work that takes considerable time to write up and publish (Wenger 1987). There may, then, be conflicts between obligations to commissioners, in terms of either quick publication, or sometimes (if the findings are politically sensitive) not publishing at all, and the demands of academic research. For Stephen Gorard (2002), 'quality' is the arbiter of these dilemmas: ethical research, he argues, is research that does not squander public money, and researchers have a responsibility to the general public (not just the participants), who may stand to benefit from any findings, to produce high-quality research with valid and reliable findings.

Conclusion

We have discussed ethical research practice as that of balancing a number of sets of responsibilities. Doing qualitative health research may generate particular ethical dilemmas, because in addition to these (sometimes conflicting) responsibilities there may be divergent expectations from health research and social research communities. Some of these conflicts have their roots in the different models of ethical principles being utilized, whether that of respect for participants as the core principle, or whether it a more instrumental one of balancing the risks and benefits of the study for participants. This means that checklists of 'good practice' are unlikely to be a sufficient guide to many of the decisions that have to be made in designing a study: they are most useful as guides to the kinds of issues that need to be considered. However, qualitative health researchers cannot take the stance that 'anything goes'. Apart from the moral responsibilities to the various stakeholders in the research process (participants, sponsors, their professional colleagues and the wider community), there are some practical reasons why any deviations from the 'good practice' checklists need very careful justification. One rather instrumental reason is that publication of findings may be very difficult if your study is not seen as ethical, and some journals will require evidence of ethical committee approval. A more public-spirited incentive is to maintain the good faith of all stakeholders in the research process, whose trust is risked by apparent breaches in good ethical practice.

KEY POINTS
- Research involves sets of (sometimes competing) responsibilities to participants, sponsors, colleagues and the wider public.
- There are different models of the proper role of research, which stress different stakeholders in the process.
- One division is between ethical models that focus on the ends (and whether these are justified by the means) and those that focus on the process (and how it can maximize the autonomy of participants).
- Ethical guidelines are a starting point for considering the ethical implications of a study. Given the diverse designs and approaches used in qualitative research, they are rarely a sufficient guide to ethical practice.
- Some key issues qualitative researchers should consider at the outset include informed consent, protecting privacy and the representation of research participants.

EXERCISES
1   For the project you designed for Exercise 3 at the end of Chapter 2, consider all of the potential stakeholders. What particular ethical responsibilities would you have to each of them in carrying out the study and disseminating the results? Do any of them conflict, and if so, how would you balance your responsibilities?

2   Imagine an ethnographer wants to come and live in your neighbourhood or work in your workplace to carry out a long-term study of health behaviours. What concerns would you have as a potential participant in this research? Outline the responsibilities you think the ethnographer has to you and your neighbours or colleagues in terms of:

(a)   confidentiality;
(b)   representing your views and behaviours;
(c)   publishing results that might be critical of your behaviours.

FURTHER READING

Homan, R. (1991) *The ethics of social research*. London: Longman. A detailed and thoughtful discussion of the issues raised by social research, rather than health research. Homan's concern is with the tendency for guidelines to restrict debate, reducing ethical decisions to a checklist, rather than encouraging debate about moral decisions.

Alderson, P. (1995) *Listening to children: children, ethics and social research*. Ilford: Barnardo's. Thought-provoking discussion of the particular issues raised by social research with young people, but many of Alderson's points are generalizable to other relatively powerless groups in the population.

Part 2

Generating and Analysing Data

4

In-depth Interviews

CHAPTER SUMMARY

Interviews are a particular kind of conversation, and are probably the most common source of qualitative data for health researchers. This chapter outlines the interactional skills interviewers need to develop, discusses the problem of language in qualitative work, particularly in cross–cultural settings, and highlights some of the practical issues interviewers need to consider, including sampling.

Introduction: terminology

The interview is the most widely used method of producing data in qualitative health research. In essence, an interview is a conversation that is directed, more or less, towards the researcher's particular needs for data. How far the researcher directs the interview, in determining the topics covered and how they are discussed, is one dimension by which research interviews could be classified. At one end of such a scale is the *structured* interview, which schedules the kind of data produced quite tightly. In this mode of interview, the interviewer must follow a specified set of questions, in a specified order, for each interview to generate comparable answers from each respondent. They are typically used in survey designs. At the other end of this scale, *informal* interviews are more like natural conversations that happen fortuitously in the field, in which data are gathered opportunistically. Perhaps the most commonly used interview types in qualitative health research are between these extremes, in the form of what are variously called *narrative*, *in-depth* or *semi-structured* interviews. In a semi-structured interview, the researcher sets the agenda in terms of the topics covered, but the interviewee's responses determine the kinds of information produced about those topics, and the relative importance of each of them. An 'in-depth' interview implies one that allows the interviewee enough time to develop their own accounts of the issues important to them. As an example, look at Case Study 8.2, which used in-depth interviews to explore how women discussed their pregnancies. In a narrative interview, the researcher's aim is to facilitate the interviewee in telling their story. The interview study described in Case Study 8.1 used narrative interviews, as a way of encouraging participants to relate the 'story' of how they came to be diagnosed with glaucoma. In practice these descriptions are used rather interchangeably, although they do suggest different emphases in terms of the amount of control the interviewer has over the encounter and what the aim of the interview is. This chapter is primarily concerned with these types of interviews, at the less structured end of the continuum, as these are properly qualitative interviews. However, many of the techniques discussed will be useful for more structured interview studies.

Developing everyday skills: what the research interview does

The research interview, as a type of interaction, has some similarities to other interactions familiar in many cultures. The job interview, the clinical history-taking, the police interrogation and the celebrity interview on television are all ways in which one party (the interviewer) attempts to produce certain kinds of data from the verbal utterances of another (the interviewee). Like these general kinds of interview, the qualitative interviewer uses their skills in social interaction to get others to disclose particular kinds of information. Most of us have developed everyday skills in social interaction that are useful in research contexts, including skills in building rapport, listening to the accounts of others, encouraging them to continue, and making people feel 'safe' to reveal their views and stories.

The qualitative research interview differs from these other kinds of interaction in that the kind of data generated are rather different. Unlike the job interview, the qualitative research interview is not 'testing' the account of the interviewee against those of others in the sample, but rather exploring their accounts, and comparing with others to develop, say, theoretical understanding of the underlying structures of beliefs. Unlike the clinical history-taking, where the health professional narrows down responses to obtain data useful for a diagnosis, the qualitative interview 'opens up' responses, and makes no a priori assumptions about the categories (such as symptoms or diagnoses) into which responses will fit. Unlike the police interrogator, the qualitative research interviewer does not assume that there is one version of the truth that can be uncovered, but that the interviewee's story will be valid as their *account* of events. By 'account' we mean the verbal report that an interviewee gives in an interview, which provides data not on their innermost feelings or beliefs (we have no access to these) but on what is said, and how it is said. In this chapter we shall develop this consideration of the aims of the qualitative research interview and the particular interactive skills needed to produce qualitative data from interviews. The first consideration is that of the nature of the data produced; that is, language data.

A word on language

In qualitative research, language is central. It is the most common form of *data* that researchers produce, first in oral form, then written as transcriptions or as excerpts in reports of qualitative work. At the same time, though, language is *method* — it is the strategy by which, through interviewing, data are produced. In qualitative work, then, language is central as both method and data, and a basic consideration is how we are to treat the language data that are produced. For language is fundamental to human understanding, to how we make sense of and shape the world around us; it is 'the most important sign system of human society' (Berger and Luckman 1967: 51). Unlike other sign systems, language is reciprocal, in that we think as we speak and think as we hear, such that in face-to-face conversations meanings are produced and reproduced in a continuous process. Through language we make sense of the world and ourselves, and then present these understandings to others. It is therefore vital that any qualitative researcher acknowledges both the theoretical and practical position accorded to 'language' in their work.

The ways in which we can think about language reflect the broad theoretical approaches to qualitative research outlined in Chapter 1. In positivist accounts, language is relatively unproblematic. It functions largely as the method of providing access to 'facts', as a window on the world, through which we can see the respondent's opinions, beliefs or behaviours. Thus in a structured interview schedule, the question 'Do you always wash your hands before cooking food?' requires a simple, one-word answer, yes or no, which acts as an indicator of a behavioural variable. To say language is not problematic in these kinds of structured schedules is not to say that it is not an important issue. Rephrasing this question as 'In what circumstances don't you wash your hands before cooking?' would presumably generate very different answers, and construct rather different accounts of hygiene behaviour. However, these considerations assume that an accurate picture of hand-washing is possible, though always potentially flawed by respondent failings. Such failings would include recall bias (problems of remembering accurately) and social desirability responses (the wish to appear as a morally worthy person to the interviewer). The interest in language in this kind of positivist approach lies in refining the language of questions to reduce such sources of bias, so that answers to questions act as the most 'accurate' indicators of behaviour possible. Sources of bias are seen as distortions to the potential of accurate representation, rather than of interest in themselves for what they tell us about the uses of language. If language is a window to the world, it is a potentially transparent one through which more or less accurate measures of human belief and behaviour can be taken, if we are careful with the linguistic prompts used.

In most qualitative work, language is more central than this. Rather than being merely a tool for gathering facts about the world, which can be sharpened to measure more accurately, language is seen as the route to understanding how the respondent sees their world (in interpretative traditions) or as the route to understanding the categories that shape the world (in more constructionist traditions). Thus, in a qualitative interview, we might be less interested in responses to a closed question ('How many times do you wash your hands before cooking?') than in *how* people talk about their hygiene behaviour in the kitchen. We might, for example, be more interested in knowing: In what contexts do they stress their attendance to hygiene? How is hygiene prioritized against other outcomes (such as practicality, or speed)? How are cleanliness and dirtiness distinguished in the kitchen, and how are these categories constructed? Thus, the language used in this kind of interview tells us about the respondent, and how they interpret, classify and represent the world. Rather than using responses as a way of indicating behaviour around the preformed category of 'hand-washing', the data the interview produces is a method for building participants' own categories of hygiene behaviour. By comparing and contrasting the accounts of interview respondents, we hope to build up a picture of the underlying cultural categories that structure individual ways of interpreting and representing such concepts as dirt, cleanliness and hygiene behaviour.

Of course, there are many other ways in which language is analysed in interview data. One tradition in sociology derives from *ethnomethodology* – the study of how people make sense of what others say and do in everyday social interaction. Here, the focus is as much on the *form* as on the content of language, and attention is paid to the ways in which social actors make sense of the world. In health research, one method associated with this approach, *con-*

versation analysis, has proved valuable in analysing talk in encounters such as those between patients and doctors. Chapter 6 discusses this as an observational method, but of course it is also possible to see the research interview as an instance of 'real' social interaction, and to pay attention to how meaning is negotiated between interviewer and respondent, as well as what content is produced (Rapley 2001).

All interviewers need to be at least aware of issues of how interaction itself produces meaning within an interview. This entails a sensitivity to the social context of the interview as experienced by both parties. It also assumes a cultural familiarity with the ways in which language is used in practice: how phrases, words and opinions are used in ways other than for their intrinsic content. As an example, consider this extract from an interview by Kathy Charmaz with a 61-year-old man who describes sharp chest pains he experienced on a walk with friends:

> [During the walk] I was white and sweating like crazy. I was in obvious pain. You didn't have to be a genius to figure out something was wrong. . . . [Later] I lay on their couch for a couple of hours while they harassed me. . . . They finally said, 'you're not going to die on my couch. Get out of here' [Laughing]. . . . I was just so sick of listening to them. I was extremely uncomfortable, and they're just at me and at me and at me like pitbull terriers or something, so I thought, 'Okay, just to shut them up'. (Charmaz 1999: 371)

Charmaz is interested in the relationships between suffering and the self in her interviewees' stories of experiencing chronic illness. She argues that suffering is a profoundly moral status, and that the placement of the speaker in 'the moral hierarchy of suffering' affects whether and how an ill person's stories will be heard. In her analysis of interview data, Charmaz points to the strategies the speaker uses for preserving self-identity, and suggests that this has a gender dimension. In the men's stories in her sample, accounts are presented to demonstrate a certain degree of bravado and risk-taking, but she also suggests that they are told in a way that asserts their claims to moral rights: 'Their stories echo with their claims to moral rights and struggles to preserve their moral status' (Charmaz 1999: 371). Thus she is using the interview data as a topic – the language as data in their own right, looking at the phrasing, the nuances, the non-verbal communications. Note how in the extract above the pauses are represented and the addition of the descriptor 'laughing' in square brackets serves to illustrate the ironic tone implied by the words used. This then is more than using the language data as simple representation of behaviour (i.e. what this person did when he thought he might be having a heart attack), but as a way of exploring the categories of risk, gender and moral status in the context of the experience of illness and suffering. This relies, though, on a sensitivity to the *ways* in which language in used, for instance in the rhetorical use of proverbial sayings, or as irony.

Language in cross-cultural settings

If language is problematic in general in qualitative research, it is of course particularly problematic where the researcher and interviewee do not share a common language. Qualitative work ideally requires fluency in the language and culture of the research setting. In anthropological fieldwork, the process of learning the language, and how different terms classify the world in the setting you are working in, is a key part of understanding the culture. Robert Pool (1994), working in Cameroon on a study originally designed to investigate reasons for the high rate of kwashiorkor (which in biomedicine is seen as resulting from protein-energy malnutrition) in one area of the country, discusses the role of interpreters. Reporting on one early discussion in the field, he notes that it was his assistant who actually conducted the 'interview', with Pool only contributing the occasional question. The discussion between him, his local assistant and the son of a local healer was carried out in English, almost as a performance for his benefit, with odd sentences in the local language, Limbum. Pool notes that in his reflections on the transcript of this discussion it became apparent how little fit there was between biomedical concepts of disease and its causes, and local accounts:

> ... the translation of illness terms seemed relatively straightforward: kwashiorkor used to be called bfaa in Limbum, nowadays it was called ngang. ... Later, however, the meanings of the words 'bfaa' and 'ngang' were to become the central focus of my research, and I was to devote hours of discussion to trying to sort out their complex and inter-linked meanings. I was also to discover that the overlap between the meanings of these terms and that of kwashiorkor was only very partial. (Pool 1994: 18–19)

Pool notes that in traditional anthropological accounts, the role of interpreters is often not discussed in detail, even when the anthropologist must have been totally reliant on them, at least in the early stages of fieldwork. He argues that his local assistant was in fact a creative part of the ethnographic enterprise, not 'an unfortunate but necessary evil distorting reality and contaminating data' (Pool 1994: 21) as they are often seen. Their competence in the local language and culture needs to be made explicit, both as facilitator of the ethnographer's data-gathering and as sounding board for exploring understandings of the local culture.

In traditional ethnography, with an extended period of fieldwork, it is at least possible to learn local languages and recruit assistants. In shorter-term research, especially if it is being conducted in a number of different cultural settings, using interpreters and translators may be a necessity. A good interpreter should be able to translate not just the literal meaning of the words used by respondents, but the contextual information also carried, such as humorous use of words and phrases, sarcasm and metaphoric use. Ideally, of course, this relies on not just bilingualism on the part of the interpreter, but biculturalism, so that meanings, rather than just words, are being translated. The interpreter must be able to understand the emotional, cultural and lexical implications of each utterance and find an equivalent in the target language. This is not an easy process. Bogusia Temple (1997), reflecting on translation issues in her work with British–Polish families, points to the (often implicit) assumptions built into particular translations, and stresses the need for open and reflexive debate about how utterances are interpreted. One example illustrates how this process of debate is part of the data analysis itself:

> My translator had written the following:
>
> 'Women can organise everything, but they cannot lead'
>
> [G]oing back to the interview, I translated as:
>
> 'Women are allowed to organise everything but to take the lead on nothing'
>
> Discussing the differences with my translator we agreed that from a word for word translation the statement could be translated either way. We discussed our views on women's position in society and discovered that they were very different [. . .] The interview meant different things to us. (Temple 1997: 616)

Through discussing with her translator the different emphasis they had put on the phrase, Temple was able to advance her own understanding of the role of Polish women in their community, and how this was seen by others (her translator) as well as herself. Thus, translation is not merely a technical service, but a vital part of the data analysis.

When translating written materials (such as survey questionnaires), best practice involves first translating into the target language, and checking this version with native speakers for comprehensibility. This version is then translated back into the source language to check that the writer's intended meaning has survived. In qualitative interview-based research this isn't possible, and there are two strategies for dealing with data collection. First, bilingual interviewers can be recruited and trained to carry out the interviews and the transcripts can be translated into the researcher's language. This of course reduces the researcher's flexibility in the data collection stage, and may mean a long delay between data collection and analysis. The alternative is simultaneous interpreting, with a bilingual interpreter used to translate each question for the interviewer, and then the respondent's answers. This requires a high degree of trust in the interpreter, who should ideally be fully involved in the study, rather than just hired for each interview. In many fieldwork settings, of course, ad hoc arrangements have to be made, and interviews may be carried out with the help of informal interpreters such as family members.

Noreen Esposito (2001) describes one strategy for managing the practicalities of translation in a study involving Spanish-speaking women in the United States. She conducted four focus groups (see Chapter 5) on women's beliefs about the menopause and their expectations of health care providers. Group interviews were facilitated by a Spanish-speaking graduate recruited from the local community who had some experience of running focus groups. She used a list of core questions developed by the research team. Esposito notes that, despite being bilingual, the facilitator was still not familiar with some of the colloquial Spanish used by participants, and that her 'communication style' was not that of the participants. In addition, the researchers recruited a trained professional translator for the group interviews, who sat in a sound-proof booth. She simultaneously verbally translated the ongoing discussion into a tape recorder into English. Once the (Spanish) tape of the research interview was also translated into English, the researchers thus had two translations available for analysis. These two tapes were, says Esposito, similar in content but had some interesting differences.

Esposito's example is of good practice when working with minority language communities in a developed country setting, with research resources including sound-proof rooms and the services of highly trained translators. She was able to use different translations to improve the validity of her data, but notes that this still restricted the kinds of qualitative analysis that could be done. Another example of using a multi-lingual research team to access views from minority language speakers is in Case Study 5.1 in the next chapter. In many settings, these kinds of resources will not be available, and it will be very difficult to find suitably skilled bilingual interpreters or researchers. Conducting an interview with an interpreter changes the social context of the interview, and the interpreter will have an influence on the data produced, just as the interviewer does. Whenever possible, interpreters (or translators of the transcript) should be fully involved in analysing the data to discuss how meanings should be analysed, and to debate the cultural implications of particular utterances. Ideally, they should not be just technical assistants, but a vital part of the research team.

Assumptions about our own language

Working with your own language does not eradicate problems of translation. To some extent all language use implies a translation, in which we assume shared meanings but cannot take them for granted. This is most explicit when interviewing those from other cultural groups, who may use particular terms in very different ways. Young people are an obvious example, as the meanings of vernacular words can change quite rapidly. The following extract, for instance, comes from a study of bilingual young people's experiences of translating for their parents in health care settings. The young people and the interviewer are fluent in English, but the interviewer (I) has to check on her understanding of an (English) term that the 16-year-old interviewees (R1 and R2) have used in relating the story of a health care encounter:

R1: I was translating for my mum, and he [the doctor] is like, screwing me as well
I: How did he do that?
R1: Just looks like [makes cross expression]
R2: A dirty look

R1: Yeah, dirty look. He most probably thought I was like cussing him because I started laughing when I was speaking to my Mum, translating, yeah, so that's probably why he started screwing me.
I: Screaming at you?
R1: Screwing me
I: Oh, screwing, is that what you said when he was staring at you, it's called screwing?
R1: Yeah

In this example, the context was enough to alert the interviewer that the young men to whom she is talking are not using the term 'screwing' in either its literal English meaning, or the slang meaning with which she was familiar (to have sex with), although she first mishears the term as 'screaming'. There are not always, though, enough clues to prompt the interviewer to check out their understanding of words and phrases in this way. Even when the use of language is apparently similar, we can't make any assumptions about shared meanings.

To some extent, the more social and cultural similarities there are between interviewer and interviewee, the more we are likely to assume shared meaning. It is much more difficult to prompt ('what do you mean by . . .') in such situations, as this implies a breach of the communality which is often the basis of rapport and trust. To interrupt too often with requests for clarification risks disrupting the ordinary flow of a story. Thus, the existence, or otherwise, of shared language or culture can have advantages and disadvantages. On the one hand, shared meanings may mean taken-for-granted aspects of daily life are not problematized, thus missing out on analytical depth. But if the interviewer is a complete 'alien', and all aspects of the encounter are problematized, there is little opportunity to develop the trust and rapport needed for successful interviewing and for collaboratively generating meaning from the encounter. However, these unintentional misunderstandings also have the potential to enhance the data and their interpretation by providing the opportunity to pursue meaning (and consequently analysis) in more depth. The example in Case Study 4.1, from Nicki Thorogood's (1988) study, in which she interviewed Afro-Caribbean women in inner London, illustrates this with examples from interviewees' responses to questions about family members.

In-depth interviews: what they can and can't do

The research interview can be seen, then, as a specific kind of interaction, in which the researcher and the interviewee produce language data about beliefs, behaviour, ways of classifying the world, or about how knowledge is categorized. These data consist of accounts of the world, not direct representations of that world. A commonly cited shortcoming of interviews is that they only provide access to what people *say*, not what they *do*. From a positivist perspective this is a problem: if we are using interviews to gather data about

Case Study 4.1   Interviewing women in London: expectations and differences

(Source: Thorogood, N. (1988) *Health and the management of daily life amongst women of Afro-Caribbean origin in Hackney,* University of London)

The project, which was part of a larger study researching minor tranquillizer use, aimed to look at a broad range of 'coping strategies' amongst a group of women. I initially introduced this as being a way in which women could help influence service improvement and policy development. This, however, seemed rather nebulous and abstract and clearly was not acting as a big incentive for women to participate. On one occasion when asking a woman to take part I simply said 'as it would help me with my education' and this (the truth) proved to be a more motivating reason (the woman agreed straight away, saying 'yes of course dear, if it will help you with your educa-tion'). This is operating on two levels; one, the appeal to education is an appeal to a discourse to which the women already subscribe; second, it acknowledges that the interviewee is the one doing the giving and this allows them the dominant role in the negotiation – they can offer you some-thing to be kind, helpful, even charitable towards you, rather than the one being 'helped' (or patronized) by potentially benefiting from the research. However, potential interviewees can also employ strategies for refusing, for example being out when you get there. In this project two women agreed to be interviewed and then gave completely plausible, but false, addresses!

As a way of drawing the interview to a close and 'winding down' from the personal level of the interview I had produced what I had believed to be a relatively straightforward 'check list of facts', asking for marital status, num-ber of children, parents' details and so on to provide a thumbnail biography of each participant. Hardly any of these categories turned out to be unpro-blematic. Many of the women had had more than one partner, several did not have full details of their biological fathers, or know where they were (UK or Caribbean, alive or dead). The 'facts' about siblings caused problems too, as many women had siblings who had one different parent. These were often all included, but the most important siblings tended to be the children of their own mothers, whilst many had fathers who had left to form other families, had run the two concurrently ('outside families') or had sim-ply had many children with other women ('outside children') of whom the interviewee was aware. Of course not all their mother's children had the same father and several of the younger women had at least one older sibling living in the Caribbean, often the child of their mother's early first pregnancy. These complexities tended to occur more often in the younger women's accounts. The older women, however, were more likely to recall siblings who had died, often including late miscarriages and still births (as they did when counting their own children). Because of my cultural predilection *not* to count these 'non-live' births, 'half-siblings' and 'step-siblings' (although 'step' was in fact a term never used), I became increasingly confused by who they were talking about and ultimately, when we filled in the 'facts' after having spent the last 4 hours or so talking about only one brother (for instance), they would then say that they had two (but one had died, or was stillborn). The practical solution to this was to move the 'check list' to the start of the interview, thus producing a kind of working 'cast list' for their story. The research outcome was to problematize my taken for granted understanding of 'family' and its meanings and to enable me to produce more informed analysis of their experiences.

Amongst the sample of younger women I was of a similar age and this gave us certain experiences in common. I think it also made being interviewed by me seem less institutional. Although some of this age group were still teenagers, perhaps my experience as a youth worker enabled us to form relationships more quickly. Surprisingly my age also seemed to be a positive factor when interviewing the older women. In these instances I was the same age as a daughter would be (in all but two cases they actually did have a daughter in her twenties). This I believe had the effect of making them feel more powerful and more in control and as if they were (as indeed they were) educating me.

people's hand-washing behaviour, our information will be 'flawed' in that accounts of the frequency of hand-washing will not necessarily bear any direct relationship to how often people really wash their hands. In terms of research design, qualitative interviews would be a poor choice of method if our aim were to investigate the rate of hand-washing in a community. This does not mean that these qualitative accounts are not valid, or that interviewees are lying. Interview data can be valid, so long as the interview is treated as a contextual account, not as a proxy representation of some other reality.

What interview data do less well is produce information about how people interact or behave in contexts other than interviews. As Silverman (1998) puts it, qualitative interview studies are 'fundamentally concerned with the environment around the phenomenon rather than the phenomenon itself'. He argues that the in-depth interview has been perhaps over-used in health research, and that more observational methods (such as analysing what actually happens in a consultation, rather than merely patients' accounts of the interaction) would often provide more useful evidence.

However, if we remember that what we are accessing in interviews are *accounts*, rather than subjective beliefs, or objective reports of behaviour, interviews are an invaluable resource. Analysing interview accounts provides data on what people say and how they say it. Given that language is the primary way in which we make sense of the world, communicate that understanding to others and (from a constructivist perspective) shape the world, interview accounts can furnish data for many research questions.

Private/public accounts

Given that accounts provided in interviews are contextual, it follows that different kinds of accounts will be provided in different interview settings.

One key factor that shapes the kind of data generated is the relationship between interviewer and interviewee. In the one-off interview, however good the interviewer is at gaining rapport, the encounter is still one of strangers, and many researchers have contrasted the accounts provided in the first interview with those later on, when the researcher is more trusted, and treated as less of a stranger. Jocelyn Cornwell (1984), in her research on the health beliefs of people in East London, contrasted what she called the 'public' accounts given by her interviewees early on in the research with the more 'private' accounts she was given in follow-up interviews. In the 'public' accounts, people were more likely to provide 'socially acceptable' views, or those that reproduced the dominant moral meanings of health in wider society. These views were more likely to be provided when the researcher was less well known, and when she was asking more general questions about health beliefs. Private views were those that may be less acceptable, more 'deviant', and that were based on real experiences. These were more likely to be revealed once the interviewer was trusted as a confidante, rather than a researcher, and in telling stories about their own experiences of health and illness. The 'private' views are not necessarily more valid than the public ones (they may, for instance, be exaggerated for dramatic effect, or to present the interviewee in a sympathetic light), but there are different contexts in which each is likely to be expressed.

In his study of parents with children with a disability, Patrick West (1990) discusses these contextual differences as one explanation for differences in findings between his own and earlier studies on the same topic. In previous research, he notes, parents reported a relatively unproblematic process of diagnosis, a good relationship with medical personnel, and relatively little disruption of family life. In his own study, based on repeated interviews with families, and with his position as separate from the hospital and other agencies, he claims to have accessed more 'private' accounts from families. These interviews generated a very different picture of how families coped with a child with a disability, and stressed the 'troubles' of coping, rather than stoic acceptance, and negative or marginal views of professionals. The differences between his and earlier accounts from the literature, argues West, reflect the different types of interview undertaken. His were from the perspective of a 'family friend' who had gained the trust of parents over time, rather than from a one-off interview, in which parents may feel they have to present the 'acceptable' image of coping parents, grateful to the professionals caring for their child. West goes on to note that this, in itself, does not mean the 'private' accounts are necessarily more valid. People may tell negative stories about medical encounters for a variety of reasons, and we cannot assume that these accounts reflect any external 'reality' of the encounter.

Stimson and Webb's (1975) study of stories about consultations in general practice, for instance, demonstrates that interviews on this topic are useful for accessing the ways in which patients 'make sense' of the encounter, but may tell us very little about what actually went on. Stories about general practitioners are, they note, a common topic of everyday conversation, and ones that invoke empathy in listeners, and a desire to cast the teller in a more active role than might actually be possible in the real encounter. It could be argued that if we are interested in the phenomenon itself (i.e. the behaviour of medical professionals) rather than just the ways in which accounts of it are utilized in everyday conversation, then interviews alone would not suffice. Patrick West used observations of out-patient appointments to validate parents' accounts of issues such as delays in communicating diagnoses and reluctance to discuss medication or psychosocial consequences.

Cultural factors and interviewing

We have suggested that the interview is a format with which most people are familiar, in that they know the broad 'rules of engagement'. These include: the interview is a setting in which it is acceptable to ask relatively personal questions, the interviewee will respond to prompts provided by the interviewer, and the interviewer (usually) will provide less information about themselves. There is a 'social role' for the interviewee, just as much as for the interviewer, and qualitative interviewing relies on all parties understanding the conventions of an interview. However, these 'rules' about the meaning of an interview cannot be assumed. In some settings the format of an interview can carry threatening connotations, or simply not be a recognized format for 'normal' social interaction. Stone and Campbell (1984), for instance, report their study of the validity of information gained from surveys of family-planning knowledge in Nepal. Although they are concerned with interviews used for structured surveys, their comments are relevant to other research settings in which the interviewer would be a relative 'stranger' to the respondents. They note that many rural Nepalese people will be unfamiliar with the survey format of questions and answers, and with the notion of 'privacy' in providing answers. In some settings, particularly in rural areas, it may be impossible to interview people without others being present, and family-planning services may be one topic that is culturally inappropriate to discuss in public. One example of the interview providing misleading data was knowledge of abortion. In the survey, villagers had been asked if they 'had heard of abortion', and about a quarter said they had not. However, the researchers knew that villagers were all aware of abortions. Within the survey interview, interviewees had interpreted the question as one of knowing about the techniques, or knowing someone who had had one. This was how the topic of 'abortion' would have been framed within the relatively 'public' context of a survey interview. Although a more sensitive wording of the question could solve some problems of this nature, Stone and Campbell maintain that the very context of a questionnaire interview is 'socially and linguistically awkward' (Stone and Campbell 1984) in this setting.

Even in cultures where there is an accepted interview format for generating information from individuals, cultural factors shape the kinds of accounts particular kinds of people can legitimately generate within it. Those being interviewed will 'place' the interviewer in terms of their institutional allegiances, presumptions about what they want to find out, and their social and cultural characteristics. There is a range of potential 'interviewee' social roles, and the placing of the interviewer will influence the one adopted. Institutional allegiances, such as whether the interviewer introduces themselves as a student, a researcher for a government department or from a university, will impact not only on willingness to be interviewed, but also the kind of person that the interviewee will present. Social, cultural and personal characteristics will inevitably shape the kind of relationship established, and how those involved frame the interaction. Characteristics such as age, gender and ethnicity cannot be eliminated, nor is it desirable that they are. Although there is some evidence that in some settings people are more willing to express less socially acceptable views to those of similar backgrounds, it should not be assumed that matching (for gender, ethnicity and so on) where possible is 'best' practice. There are likely to be advantages in terms of access and establishment of rapport, but possibly disadvantages in terms of assumptions of shared meanings, and possibly (especially in relatively small sub-groups) distrust of confidentiality. Instead, the researcher must account for the interplay between the social positions of the actors involved in the data generated, as this in itself is part of the data.

A qualitative methodology foregrounds the subjective experience of the participants, but it cannot be presumed that the interviewer is simply a conduit for the expression of those experiences. Similarities and differences both in aspects of social identity and experience and in social power will clearly have a major impact on the social encounter that is 'the interview', and shape which particular experiences interviewees choose to discuss, and how they talk about them. Early discussions of the impact and ethical dilemmas produced by this were raised by sociologists exploring implications of feminist methodology for research practice (Oakley 1981; Finch 1984; Smith 1988). Their resolution of the dilemma was that participants should be the subjects rather than the objects of the research, and that rather than pursuing the quantitative goal of eliminating difference (or bias), social differences in the interview relationship should be acknowledged and included in the analytical frame. This perspective has been influential in qualitative methodology more generally, with the acceptance that social differences and similarities between researcher and researched should be acknowledged, documented and accounted for in the analysis. Examining the salience of, for instance, differences and similarities with respect to ethnicity when talking about aspects of health is a useful way of identifying how ethnic identity may contribute to the ways in which people account for their health.

Social differences in interviews

Social differences between interviewer and interviewee can exist in relation to nationality, race, class, socio-economic status, age and gender. The impact of social 'difference' on the data produced in research is complex. As Rosalind Edwards notes: 'race does not simply exist as an object of study or a variable in analysis, it enters into the research process itself . . . and importantly influences the relationship with those we are researching' (Edwards 1990: 482). This applies, of course, to other dimensions of social difference (and similarity).

From a feminist perspective, Rosalind Edwards (1990) notes that, as a white woman interviewing Afro-Caribbean women in Britain, race framed the whole process of her interviews, from gaining access to potential interviewees to the establishment of a trusting relationship in the interview itself. She found that, rather than assuming a commonality based on gender, interviewees were distrustful because of her different structural position in society. Many areas, such as details about family life, could only be addressed in interviews after she had acknowledged this different position, rather than assuming a similarity, as she did with interviewees of the same gender and ethnicity. However, Edwards did not see these factors as 'barriers' to be overcome in carrying out her research, but rather as data that helped her understand the ways in which gender and ethnic roles were experienced, and which aspects of identity are prioritized in different relationships. In contrast, Penelope Scott (1999), in her experience of researching white British and Caribbean people with diabetes, notes how her Caribbean background facilitated a level of trust and rapport, evidenced in the personal stories told and the hospitality extended, with the Caribbean interviewees. This was not evident in most of the interviews with the white British participants, which were in general shorter and less likely to cover personal details. Scott suggests that a dichotomy of 'public' and 'private' views may not capture the diverse ways in which different groups will respond to the experience of being interviewed.

In more positivist research traditions, the problem of these differences is one of attempting to eliminate potential sources of bias. In qualitative research, though, there is more typically an acceptance that *any* interview account is situated and contextual, and that we therefore have to account explicitly for the ways in which social and cultural characteristics have an impact on the kind of data collected. For Edwards and Scott, who were interviewing people with both social similarities (of gender) and differences (of ethnicity), this was facilitated by an analytical awareness of the different kinds of data produced across their interviews. Other possibilities are using comparisons between the data collected by different interviewers within one project as an aid to thinking about the interplay of social identities and accounts of experience, or comparing your own findings with those of other researchers (as Patrick West did in his study of parents with children with disabilities).

'Elite' interviewing

Much of the textbook advice on interviewing assumes that the researcher is in a relatively powerful position vis-à-vis the interviewee, and that methodological and ethical problems relate to offsetting this imbalance. However, many health research studies, especially those of policy development or implementation, involve interviews with those who are relatively more powerful than the interviewer. Interviewing senior civil servants, clinicians or health service managers presents somewhat different problems of 'cultural difference' if the interviewer is a student, or a less powerful health profes- sional. First, many respondents in these 'elite' groups will be difficult to recruit to an interview study, if invited in their professional role, and may offer only brief appointments for the interview (see Case Study 4.2, below). Second, in brief interviews, managers or policy advisers will be speaking 'for their organization', and the public accounts you generate may have been more efficiently gathered from official documents or written replies. If the aim is to gather the less official accounts of, for instance, how policy is made or implemented, methods other than in-depth interviewing may be needed, such as observation of meetings.

However, interviewing elite respondents may be the only method for acces- sing certain kinds of data. Renée Danziger, in her comparative study of HIV testing policies in Britain, Sweden and Hungary (Danziger 1998), characterized her interview method as 'elite interviewing' (Dexter 1970), as the data were gathered from civil servants, academics, directors of voluntary organizations and public health specialists. Her justification for using interview data is that in many countries (including Britain and Sweden) there was no official 'HIV testing policy' that could be identified in official documents. Such policies had to be pieced together from a variety of sources, including government and health service directives and the accounts of key informants. Danziger's interviews with policy-makers and academics provided her with access to the kinds of cultural beliefs that underpinned HIV testing policies in the three countries, and contributed to her discussion of how different policies might be culturally appropriate in different settings.

Techniques: developing interview skills

Given the fact that the data generated from an interview are the product of the specific interaction of that interview, and that there is need for sensitivity around social norms of 'interviewing' in particular localities, it is of course impossible to provide a general list of rules for 'good technique'. The key to developing research interview skills is to consider carefully the aims of the interview (Is it to generate stories? To elucidate a broad range of views? To explore how people talk about an issue?), and to identify how these are achieved within 'normal' interaction in the setting within which you are working and how they are likely to be achieved in an interview. The process of identifying the necessary skills is of course data in itself, as you learn how to ask questions and what kinds of topics are discussed in particular settings, and how they are dealt with. A good way of developing skills is to look carefully at early transcripts with a critical eye on interview techniques and ask questions such as:

- Did you interrupt when the interviewee was still speaking?
- Could you have left longer gaps for them to continue speaking?
- Were there points at which you could have prompted for more information?
- Did your questions appear judgemental, or too inquisitive, or leading?

The following sections outline some of the practical considerations for planning and conducting interview studies to help think through what might work best, given the aims of the study, the kind of data you hope to generate from the interviews, and the setting.

Access

How does a researcher get people to agree to be interviewed? In some cases there is a legitimacy acquired from being part of a clinical setting – if the doctor asks if you would like to take part a patient may find it difficult to refuse, and indeed may feel that if the doctor thinks it is a good idea then it must be. Often 'key informants' are used as a means of gaining access to a more general population; thus the organizer of a pensioners' luncheon club, or the leader of a leisure club, may agree to ask (or to let you ask) other members to participate. The interview relationship depends on a certain amount of mutual trust and obligation. The most difficult interviews are those done with no introduction (cold calling), since the research and the interviewer have no external legitimacy to call on. In such cases the interviewer has to 'sell' the research – sometimes through offering small incentives (such as vouchers) or by putting a particular 'spin' on it; that is, presenting it in a way that makes it appear particularly useful, appealing or beneficial to the participant. As the example in Case Study 4.1 illustrates, for studies conducted as part of a research degree, being honest about the educative purpose of the study to the researcher may often be a good way to invite participation.

Given the particular problems of 'elite interviewing' outlined above, access to professionals can sometimes be particularly challenging. Chris Ntau's (2002) description of the process of accessing doctors in Botswana in Case Study 4.2 is perhaps typical of the experiences of many researchers.

Setting

The setting of an interview impacts on the kind of data generated (Green and Hart 1999). The same person may stress different aspects of their identity in an out-patient clinic, a private room in their home or in their workplace. In general, in most developed country settings it is easiest to interview in a private space that the interviewee feels is 'theirs'. Of course in many settings, especially in rural villages in developing countries, such privacy may be

Case Study 4.2   Problems of access in a study of doctors in Botswana

(Source: Ntau, C.G. (2002) 'Medical careers of Botswana doctors' (Report from the Phil Strong Prize), *Medical Sociology News*, 28(3): 9–12)

Chris Ntau carried out his PhD study on the medical careers of Botswana doctors. In Botswana, the migration of skilled health care workers out of the country has led to considerable pressures on the public system. His study aimed to explore the factors that influence doctors' decisions to leave by interviewing those in the public and private sectors. He discusses some of the challenges faced in getting permission to carry out the study and accessing interviewees:

> Interviewing doctors was a multistage process, involving a number of players before the interview could actually take place. The first stage started with the Office of the President, seeking a research permit. A quick response from the Office of the President gave me a false belief that things ahead would be smooth. Although obtaining the research permit was quick, more hurdles lay ahead. More permissions were required to actually start interviewing the respondents. The second stage involved requesting permission from the participating hospitals. Delays were experienced at this stage as officials took their time to respond. In one case, a response came after three months, following a series of phone calls.
>
> Once permission was granted by participating institutions, the next stage was to speak to doctors, and agree on the appointment date. A phone call to the hospital led to the hospital receptionist, who then put the researcher through to the doctor. On a bad day, it was normal to wait a long period before getting through to the doctors. On getting hold of the doctor, I quickly introduced myself, emphasizing that I was studying at a foreign university. Naming the university was helpful, in terms of getting some doctors' co-operation, as all of them had studied outside the country. The research purpose was explained and then an invitation extended to a doctor to participate. Guided by the doctor's schedule, an appointment date would then be agreed, which was by no means a guarantee that an interview would actually take place.
>
> On the agreed day, if an interview was scheduled in the afternoon, a morning reminding call was important. If the interview was in the morning, one-day advance reminder was sufficient. Cancellations and postponements were the norm, especially with doctors employed in government institutions and government officials. Reasons ranged from 'I was "on call" last night, so, I wouldn't make it today', or 'he/she is in theatre', to 'still seeing patients'. Undoubtedly, interviewing doctors, especially in conditions where they are too few, or facilities are seriously understaffed, requires a lot of patience. However, once interviews were underway, doctors readily opened up, and 'told their stories' of the 'joys' and 'hurts' of the medical profession. (Ntau 2002: 10–11)

impossible, or at least a suspicious request. On a more practical level, interviewing someone in 'their' space, particularly their home, can seem very intrusive. You are invited in but then cannot behave according to the social rules for guests, as you may have to move furniture in order to be near enough to the microphone, ask them to turn off televisions or radios in the room, or ask others to leave. A quiet room away from other distractions is ideal, but in practice it is not always possible. For example, the interviewee may have small children in their care. Few young children will be able to resist touching the equipment (with a variety of outcomes) or, if still at 'toddler stage', doing noisy 'drumming' on furniture nearby, thus obscuring huge passages of dialogue. Even other adults can turn out to be unexpectedly noisy. The tape of an interview records all the background noises that you 'screen out' whilst actually participating in it. It can seem quite rude to ask someone to turn their TV or radio off (and not very conducive to establishing rapport when you have only just entered their house), but even low-level background TV or radio results in a tape interspersed by, for instance, regular 'jingles'. Worse still are chiming clocks, particularly those that chime on the quarter-hour with 'Big Ben' chimes. Traffic noise if you are interviewing near an open window can be disruptive. Thorogood's most dramatic experience was of interviewing a young woman in her own flat which she had not been able to furnish very fully, therefore the floors and walls were bare and 'echoey'. She did, however, own a talking parrot which would pipe up every now and again during the interview. Although it did not cause any problem at the time, on replaying the tape for transcription, the noise had totally obscured parts of the interviewee's responses. When asking if she smoked at all, all you could hear on the tape was the parrot squawking 'no!' In effect, then, she had interviewed a parrot!

Rapport

Building a sense of trust with the interviewee involves presenting yourself as both non-judgemental and interested. Avoid questions, prompts and expressions that suggest disapproval or disagreement. An introduction to the interview should include your own name, the aims of the interview, a reminder that the interviewee can stop at any time, and an opportunity for them to ask questions. It is often easiest to begin the interview with a very general, open kind of question. These could be:

- 'Can you tell me what your health was like as a child?'
- 'Can you tell me what it's been like having diabetes?'
- 'Can you tell me about the kind of treatment you've had so far?'

These are really inviting the interviewee to tell something of 'their story', which immediately implies it is both a valid and interesting viewpoint to hold and express.

The topic guide and phrasing questions

These principles should also inform the kinds of questions that form the main body of the interview. Open questions, rather than closed ones inviting a 'yes' or 'no' response, are more likely to facilitate the interviewee telling their story. Qualitative interviews generally use a 'topic guide' rather than a predetermined list of questions. This can be used to orientate the interviewer to the areas to cover, and in larger studies with several interviewers can ensure that all interviews cover the same topics.

It is also useful to think of some ways of phrasing questions or generating stories, and to consider some alternatives to use when these don't work well. Avoid simply asking respondents your research question, or to reflect on your objectives. If, for instance, the research topic is 'What are the barriers to implementing evidence-based practice for surgeons?', asking a sample of surgeons the question 'What do you think about the barriers to you implementing evidence-based practice?' is likely to generate data about their 'opinions' on barriers (a rather different research question). More useful data may come from questions designed to generate accounts of how surgeons do use evidence in their working lives. This links to the discussion of qualitative research design in Chapter 2, and is essentially a matter of thinking through the phenomenon in which you are interested and how to access knowledge about that phenomenon. Thus, if the topic of interest is a narrowly based interpretation of evidence (the latest evidence based on RCTs), ask about access to these and how they are used. If the topic is broader, and relates to how evidence is used in practice, then ask about this using prompts to allow surgeons to tell their story, from their perspective. Thus, the topic guide might start with general questions about their work and move on to how they obtain evidence to inform that work and finally ask directly about 'barriers' to the use of the kinds of evidence in which you are interested.

There are a number of alternatives to straightforward questions asking about respondents' beliefs or practices. Some are listed in Box 4.1. The key issue is perhaps a flexible approach to the framing of questions, and close attention to the early interviews to assess what has worked well and what less well.

Body language

In many cultures, maintaining eye contact implies interest and active listening. However, interviewers do need to be careful about local cultural and social norms around body language. In most settings, for instance, it would be inappropriate to physically touch the interviewee except for shaking hands, but there are situations where not to do so would be unnecessarily cold. It is also important to retain an 'active listening posture', which usually involves sitting forward in one's chair, keeping your body turned towards the speaker,

---

Box 4.1   Alternatives to direct questions for interviews

- *Verbal diaries*. Ask interviewees to describe a typical day, or hospital visit, or work shift. These kinds of questions are particularly useful for early data collection, or studies where the main aim is to understand the world-view of a group of respondents. Accounts of a 'day in the life' or a particular event provide some access to what respondents think is particularly important to report, and a general 'feel' for their world, as well as presenting opportunities to probe the areas of particular interest for the study.
- Asking about '*critical incidents*' such as worst or best experiences of care. This is a useful way of uncovering what the common features of, for instance, 'good' and 'bad' care might be from patients' perspectives. Equally, professionals can be asked which kinds of clients they most like/least like dealing with, or about the most satisfying or the most difficult work situations.
- Using *vignettes* based on case studies to access normative responses. This can be particularly useful for sensitive topics, as rather than asking interviewees to reflect on their own experiences, they are asked about fictional others. They are also useful for grounding discussion in concrete cases rather than abstract 'views'. Lindsay Prior and colleagues used vignettes to explore how Cantonese speakers in England referred to traditional and Western concepts of health and illness (Prior et al. 2000). These vignettes were summary descriptions such as 'Three month old baby with vomiting, diarrhoea and high temperature' and 'Man aged 45 with dizziness, headaches and blurred vision'. They were used to prompt discussion around what problems required help and what kind of help was appropriate.
- Using *visual cues*, such as photographs or objects, to aid discussion. Gillian Bendelow (1993), for instance, used a variety of visual images, such as paintings and photographs, to prompt her interviewees to talk about pain. On topics like this, which may be difficult for many people to verbalize, visual cues can be a useful way of generating data.
- Using *visual imagery* as an aid to data collection. Asking respondents to draw, for instance, a map of their neighbourhood is a useful prompt for talking about the significance of local spaces and their health impacts. Many studies with younger children invite them to draw as well as talk, for example asking them to 'draw healthy food' or 'things that are bad for your health'.

---

nodding for both agreement and encouragement and NOT looking at your watch! This can, however, be enormously difficult to do as the interviewer is simultaneously having to worry about whether the tape is still running/recording/about to run out, nod encouragingly and meet the interviewee's eye, not to mention planning the following question or link to another unexplored area of interest.

Using prompts and probes

If the aim is to allow the interviewee to tell their story, or to provide detailed accounts of their experiences, the interviewer has to provide a facilitative audience for the story. This will usually include:

- not interrupting;
- allowing silences;
- prompts, which include the noises we make to encourage people to continue (uh-huh, mm) and the non-verbal cues such as head-nodding;
- probes, to encourage elaboration, including questions such as 'anything else?', 'and then what happened?';
- avoiding 'leading' questions that suggest a particular answer, or frame the respondents' replies for them.

In summary, qualitative interviewing relies on skills most of us have as part of our repertoire of social skills, and they can be developed through practice and sensitivity to local norms of social interaction. However, interviews are a particular kind of interaction, and careful reflexive practice is needed to ensure that the personal styles we bring to the interview are appropriate for the setting, likely to establish rapport, and likely to generate the kind of data we need for the study. Like body language, this does differ across cultures: for instance, long silences may be interpreted as aggressive, rather than facilitative, in some cultures (Simon Lewin, personal communication).

Improving reliability

Interacting and facilitating a research interview can be hard work, and it is generally difficult to write down responses while maintaining eye contact, listening, providing encouragement and planning the prompt, probe or link to the next topic of interest. In addition, few interviewers have shorthand skills to take down exactly what is said. Ideally, then, interviews should be recorded on audio-tape. It is a useful exercise to compare handwritten notes of an interview with a transcript of a tape of the same interview. Most researchers find that they missed what turn out to be the key issues, quote phrases that were never said, and mistake their own utterances for those of the interviewee in the notes taken by hand. An accurately transcribed audio-tape is the most reliable record of an interview. It can also easily be reproduced if there are several researchers involved in the project, and can be (if there is permission from research participants and the data are suitably anonymized) archived for future analysis in other studies.

However, it is not always possible to tape interviews. Some individuals will prefer not to be recorded, and in some cultures it can be a threatening request. Also, opportunistic interviews, done in the course of fieldwork, are unlikely to be taped. It is important, then, also to improve both skills in note-taking and the ability to write notes while listening actively.

If possible, it is worth investing in a good-quality tape recorder and micro-phone, as poor-quality tapes are difficult to transcribe accurately. Transcription is time-consuming, taking six to eight hours to transcribe one hour of inter-view, and the time or cost must be considered in planning the study. Some researchers prefer to transcribe all their own tapes, as this is a useful way of beginning to familiarize yourself with the data. It is certainly good practice to transcribe at least the first few yourself.

Transcribing interviews

Transcribing audio-taped conversations is of course a translation process in itself. The choices of punctuation, spelling and detail of the transcript all affect how it is read by those analysing it. For those interested in conversation analysis, there are detailed conventions to record such nuances of talk as stress, pauses of various lengths, rising and falling intonation and non-verbal noises (see ten Have 1999). For most qualitative research, such detailed transcriptions are not needed, but it is important to reproduce reliably the precise words used by the interviewee, including slang words, stutters, hesitations and interrup-tions. Everyday conversation is rarely grammatical, or conducted in complete sentences, and transcriptions should reproduce the 'actual' talk rather than a tidied-up version. The important issue is that conventions used for transcrip-tion are agreed within the project team and whoever is transcribing data. One possible set is suggested in Box 4.2. For ease of use when analysing, transcrip-tions should be printed with wide margins, numbered lines and each new speaker on a new line. To ensure confidentiality for respondents, it is a good idea to remove any identifiers, such as names or specific locations, before transcripts are used.

Box 4.2   Suggested transcript conventions

I	Start of each new utterance by interviewer
R	Start of each new utterance by respondent
?	Beginning of utterance by unidentified speaker
wo-	Word interrupted by next utterance
(word)	Word(s) in round brackets indicate transcriber's guess at an unclear word
CAPITALS	Words spoken more loudly than others
(. . .)	Indicate unclear material omitted by transcriber

In extracts reported in papers and reports:

[ ]	Square brackets enclose material added by author
. . .	Indicate material omitted by author

Sampling: how many and who to interview?

Perhaps the most common question from novice researchers is 'How many interviews do I need to do?' In quantitative work the answer can be calculated if you know something about the population, and the level of confidence you want in any differences found not being due to chance. The aim in quantitative studies is to produce a sample that is representative in a statistical way of the whole population of interest, and some kind of *probability sample*, in which each member of the population has an equal chance of being selected, is usually used. In qualitative work there are typically other considerations, and the sample size for an interview study depends on the aims – what you are expecting the data to do in terms of answering a question. As we have seen, in a case study such as a life history a sample size of one may be quite adequate, if the aim is to explore a deviant case or the subjective experience of one illustrative individual. For some studies, sampling decisions have to be made opportunistically, if there are few potential interviewees who may be willing to agree. In general, though, most qualitative research has an aim of *purposive* (sometimes called purposeful) *sampling*; that is, explicitly selecting interviewees who it is intended will generate appropriate data.

Patton (1990) suggests that the overall aim of purposive, as opposed to probability, sampling is to include 'information-rich cases for in-depth study' (Patton 1990: 182). To achieve this, a number of different sampling strategies are possible. These include: extreme or deviant case sampling, typical case sampling, and snowball sampling. Another interesting strategy suggested is 'political sampling', or taking into account the political considerations that apply to both sample size and selection. Patton (1990: 180) suggests that choosing politically important cases is one strategy for improving the chances of a project gaining attention and the findings being used. Thus, if evaluating a nation-wide health service reorganization, it may be possible to select case studies in high-profile hospitals to maximize the chance of media interest. Equally, such considerations will suggest not selecting high-profile cases if the findings are likely to be sensitive and such interest will be counterproductive. Less obvious political issues also influence sampling strategies. For qualitative findings to be credible for those likely to be using the results, it may be important to choose respondents from a range that they would identify as 'representative'. Thus, if researching the views of cancer patients on information needs, it might be important to include patients from a range of social classes and localities and with different diagnoses so that oncologists are less likely to dismiss the findings as irrelevant to their practice, even if there is no theoretical justification for choosing these groups of patients. Thus one practical answer to 'How many people should I interview?' is 'However many will be credible to the users of your research'.

A more methodological answer to sample size is implied by a grounded theory approach (see Chapter 8). This approach advocates *theoretical sampling*, or including interviewees (or the 'events and incidents' that interviewees and other sources provide) in the sample on the basis of both an understanding of the field, emerging hypotheses from ongoing data analysis, and a deliberate attempt to 'test' such hypotheses. The intention is to keep sampling and analysing data until nothing new is being generated. This point is called 'saturation' and the strategy is 'sampling to saturation'. Although initial decisions about sites and areas of interest have to be taken, and thought through very carefully, theoretical sampling involves a flexible approach that is to a large extent dependent on ongoing data analysis, which generates new conceptual ideas to test against primary data. Strauss and Corbin (1990: 181–93) discuss a three-stage sampling strategy in which the early stages are relatively indiscriminate, because the researcher has little idea of which concepts are going to be theoretically relevant. A *convenience sample* would be sufficient at this point, and opportunistic interviews (for instance, informal interviews with those in the field) may be rich sources of data. As data analysis proceeds, the researcher deliberately seeks to include those who are likely to generate data of more relevance to the concepts that are emerging as important. Finally, in the later stages of a study, sampling will be more discriminating, and intended to test the emerging theories, by for instance deliberately seeking out deviant cases or to test how well hypotheses hold up in different settings.

In principle, the methodological justification for theoretical sampling is convincing and it offers a rigorous way of ensuring thorough data collection. However, there are a number of practical difficulties. First, in funded work few researchers have the kind of resources that allow the relatively open-ended commitment to data collection that theoretical sampling implies. We are likely to run out of time or money before 'saturation' has happened. Second, most sponsors of research will want a more or less detailed account of exactly who, and how many, will be interviewed within the protocol before research is funded. The same may apply to ethics committees (see Chapter 3), who may need to know precisely which population groups are being sampled. If each new category of interviewee has to be approved by an ethics committee as they are theoretically sampled, this becomes cumbersome to manage. Third, the point of 'saturation', in the sense intended by grounded theory, relates not merely to 'no new ideas coming out of the data' but to the notion of a conceptually dense theoretical account of the field of interest in which all categories are fully accounted for, the variations within them explained, and all relationships between the categories established, tested and validated for a range of settings. This process is potentially limitless, and the point at which 'saturation' has happened is perhaps more contentious than Strauss and Corbin imply. Certainly the phrase 'theoretical saturation was reached' has become rather a routine disclaimer in many journal articles of fairly thin analysis, with little evidence of the kind of density of theory intended by Strauss and Corbin.

If 'saturation' is not a practical answer to the question of sample size for most applied health researchers, it does perhaps suggest one. If addressing a fairly specific research question, the experience of most qualitative researchers is that in interview studies little 'new' comes out of transcripts after you have interviewed twenty or so people in one 'category'. To illustrate, in a study of bilingual children's experiences of interpreting for their families in health care settings (Green et al. 2002a), we were interested in including people from a range of more settled and more recently arrived communities, including both young men and young women and including those who lived in areas where lots of other young people spoke the same language as well as those who were more isolated from others in the same community. The aims were both to sample a representative group of young people, in terms of the range of issues suggested in the literature as important to how people perceive their language use, and to explore how social and cultural differences might shape experience. We thus proposed a sampling strategy that included 15 young people from *each of* four different language communities, and aimed to recruit both males and females within each group. We then identified established community groups (such as youth clubs and homework clubs) in areas that were socially mixed in terms of linguistic communities living there, and some that were more homogeneous. The total sample size was therefore 60, but within that were various sub-samples, such as 30 young women, 15 Vietnamese speakers, 40 young people born outside the UK, 20 who were the only person who spoke their 'mother tongue' in their school class. This example illustrates the kinds of mixed sampling strategies that are used in practice to generate information-rich cases. Although 'theoretically sampled' in terms of the kinds of cultural variables likely to be important analytically, the sample was also a convenience sample to the extent that the actual young people invited to take part were those attending the community facilities sampled when we were doing fieldwork.

Conclusion

Interviews are the mainstay of much qualitative health research. The limitations of interviews as a source of data have been noted: they only provide access to what people say, not what they do; the accounts we collect are a reflection of the interview context, not any 'essential' truth about respondents' beliefs; the analysis of interview data relies on considerable local cultural as well as linguistic knowledge. However, they are a relatively efficient way of generating data on almost all health topics. Their strengths lie in appropriate use: when the research question requires analysis of accounts, and when the researcher is reflexive about how the research context impacts on the data collected. Good interviewing skills rely on sensitive use of local cultural norms of social interaction. The development of appropriate interview protocols and techniques for a particular project is thus an essential element of good research practice, but is also part of the data collection itself. The example of how to deal with the questions about respondents' biographical details in Case Study 4.1 illustrates this: Thorogood's decision to put the questions at the beginning of the interview 'worked better', but the process of discovering why her questions didn't work at the end of the interview provided valuable data about how her interviewees categorized family relationships.

KEY POINTS

- The qualitative research interview is a particular kind of social interaction, which is recognized in most Western settings, but may be less familiar in other settings.
- The status of interview data depends on the epistemological underpinning of the study.
- Using interpreters in qualitative work is particularly problematic. When used, they should be an integral part of the research team.
- Qualitative research requires reflexivity about how the setting and social characteristics of the interviewer affect the data produced.

EXERCISES

1 The best practice for in-depth interviewing is to carry one out. There is nothing quite like having first-hand experience of trying to juggle all the various social and environmental factors, thinking about the next question, and trying to decide how far to pursue a particular strand whilst still trying to keep focused on the actual spoken exchanges! If possible, identify a volunteer you do not know well to carry out a practice in-depth interview on a relatively neutral topic such as 'Experiences of dental care' or 'Preventing accidental injury'. Identify your aims for the interview (do you want to encourage narrative accounts of, say, experiences of accidental injury, or to identify health beliefs about dental hygiene?). Think of a number of prompts, and use some of the suggestions in Box 4.1 to frame some questions. After the interview, get your interviewee to give you feedback on whether you succeeded in putting them at ease, and whether they felt they covered the issues that were relevant to them on the topic.

2 If it is inappropriate or impossible to do your own interview, many insights can be gained from paying attention to the detail of interviews in other settings. Students may have access to television, radio, newspaper or magazine interviews with a variety of 'respondents': these may be politicians, experts, lay campaigners, media celebrities or simply members of the general public. Select one or more of these interviews for analysis and then watch, listen to or read them with the following in mind:

- How does the setting influence the content or manner of the interview?
- How does the 'world-view' (epistemological position) of the interviewer or interviewee affect their questions or response? Is this position implicit or explicit?
- How is the main topic of the interview approached?
- Do certain types or styles of question produce different answers?

- What particular aspects of replies are explored further? How is this done?
- In a political interview, for example, this may be by challenging the interviewee, which one would not normally expect in a social research interview. What effect does this have? How might it be approached differently?

Interviews of these types are in many ways very different from a social research interview. There are, however, many points of similarity. In the absence of the 'real thing', a great deal of insight and knowledge can be gained by the close observation of 'interview technique' more generally.

FURTHER READING

Patton, M.Q. (1990) 'Qualitative interviewing', in *Qualitative evaluation and research methods* (2nd ed.). Newbury Park, CA: Sage, pp. 299–368. This has detailed and practical information on how to design better prompts and questions in qualitative work, and some very useful suggestions for different ways of asking for information and views from respondents.

5

Group Interviews

CHAPTER SUMMARY

Group interviews have the advantage over one-to-one interviews of providing access to interaction between participants, and thus some insight into how social knowledge is produced. In addition, they can be a useful way of researching some sensitive issues, such as dissatisfaction with services. In health research they have been used widely in health promotion, health services research and in needs assessment. Different types of group interview are discussed, including focus groups and natural groups.

Introduction

By 'group interviews' we mean any interview in which the researcher simultaneously gathers data from more than one participant. These range from opportunistic interviews held with small, naturally occurring groups during fieldwork to specially recruited focus groups gathered together purely for research purposes. In developed country settings, focus groups have become a widely used technique for gathering data to inform needs assessment, evaluate services and conduct research on group norms. In developing countries, community meetings are often used for data-gathering, as part of a participatory approach to set research agenda and in programme evaluation. What these various data collection formats have in common is that, unlike the one-to-one interview, they provide access to how people interact with each other as well as with a researcher.

Different kinds of group interview: an overview

The term 'focus group' is often used in the literature to describe any formal group interview. However, there are a number of more or less formal ways in which social researchers use data collected from groups, rather than individuals, and it may be useful to begin by distinguishing different kinds of groups used in research. Jeannine Coreil (1995) has suggested a typology (outlined in Box 5.1) based on sampling strategy and aims. These are, of course, 'ideal types', and any particular interview might have elements of more than one type, but they are a helpful way of orientating us to the variety of aims researchers might have in conducting group interviews.

The type of group interview chosen will depend on the aim of the study and feasibility. If the aim is to generate 'naturalistic' data, then pre-existing 'natural' groups may be the format of choice, whereas selected focus groups would be more appropriate if a wide range of views across the population was needed. The setting will also influence the format. Coreil notes that in research in rural areas of developing countries, the lack of a meeting room means that in practice any group interview may involve a shifting group, as people (and even animals!) drift in and out of the room or space in which the interview is taking place. In many research settings privacy may not be possible, and group interviews may be used simply because it is not possible to talk to people individually. This chapter is concerned primarily with the methodological and practical issues raised by using focus groups or natural groups to gather data for qualitative health research, but as the other two formats in Coreil's typology (consensus panels and community interviews) are sometimes used in qualitative health research, we shall describe them briefly.

Consensus panels

Consensus panels are groups gathered to come to some agreement about an issue, such as priorities for health care spending, an agenda for health research, or guidelines for clinical practice (Murphy et al. 1998). Though not strictly an

Box 5.1 Coreil's typology of group interviews

Interview type	Features	Typical uses
Consensus panel	Often composed of key informants or experts Seeks group consensus or normative reactions More narrow, closed-ended stimulus material	Agreeing clinical protocols, resource prioritization
Focus group	Participants selected to meet sampling criteria Seeks broad range of ideas of open-ended topic Formal, controlled pre-arranged time and place Usually audio-taped and transcribed for analysis	Testing health promotion materials, exploring service users' views
Natural group	Group exists independently of the research study Format formal or informal Interview guide loosely followed Usually recorded by written notes	Ethnographic data collection (informal), social research (formal)
Community interview	Open to all or large segments of a community Usually recorded by written notes	Project planning, programme evaluation

Source: Adapted from Coreil (1995).

interview method, they are sometimes used in qualitative studies, and to help set research agenda (see, for instance, Bond and Bond 1982) as well as to inform planning. There are a number of different formal methods for reaching decisions, such as:

- *Delphi groups.* In Delphi groups the participants do not meet, but are mailed a questionnaire to invite views on the given topic. Summaries of the views of the group are then mailed back, with participants invited to change their responses in the light of the views of the group. This can be repeated several times, until members of the group come to a consensus.
- *Nominal group technique.* This was developed to enable groups of people with interest or expertise in an area to generate and rank ideas. The group is 'nominal' because it is a group only in name, and does not necessarily exist for other purposes. The structure is highly controlled to reduce the effects of dominating

members. Each participant privately and independently writes their comments on the group's question. These are all then listed and discussed. Each participant then ranks their top ten ideas, with those with most votes listed and discussed. Finally, points are awarded to the top ten ideas to rank them. Gallagher et al. (1993), for instance, used nominal groups to explore patient and professional views about diabetic care. Nominal groups of experts, generalist professionals, patients and carers were brought together to address the question 'What things are important in making people satisfied with diabetes care?' Qualitative analysis of the discussion was used to explore the reasons for differences in how people ranked aspects of care, and Gallagher et al. claim that the technique is a useful research tool, especially in exploratory work.

- *Consensus conferences.* This is a generic term for workshops or discussion groups where participants come to some consensus through debate and interaction. Some aim to empower participants in addition to developing consensus (see Rowe and Frewer 2000 for a review). Citizens' juries are one such approach, where representative members of the public are invited to hear from experts, ask questions and discuss possible policy options. They are increasingly used, largely in developed country settings, as a way of including public views in policy development (see, for instance, Cosby et al. 1986; Lenaghan 1999). Consensus conferences are also used to involve professionals in such activities as guideline development (see Murphy et al. 1998).

Community interviews and participatory methods

Participatory methods aim to redress the unequal power relationships inherent in research such that researchers share responsibility and knowledge with participants. Built on democratic principles, the intention is that communities will determine the research agenda, and participate in the process of research, action and development. Community interviews are a key plank in this kind of action research, as a route to developing participatory practice rather than merely gathering data. Development projects often rely on community meetings at the outset to generate interest in the project, answer questions from the community and include community priorities in the research agenda. As an example, look at the way in which workshops were used in the Stepping Stones project described in Case Study 2.2 to identify community priorities. Often these are not seen as part of the formal data collection process, although they may generate useful information. In other cases, community interviews are included as an essential element of gathering data and attempting a more democratic style of research. Rachel Baker and Rachel Hinton (1999), for instance, discuss their use of group interviews in their work on street children and refugee families in Nepal. Both were concerned to work with participants' own agendas for health and well-being. For them, group interviews were both 'an exploratory tool to illuminate issues of concern within the community' (Baker and Hinton 1999: 82) and 'to verify (or challenge) problems identified by the organizations, the community and the researchers' prior findings' (ibid.:

83). They discuss the potential for group work to meet the needs of researchers and communities throughout the process of participatory work. One example was street children asking Baker to facilitate skills training to enable them to find employment, something that both involved sharing knowledge and met the research aims. There are, though, limitations to how far participants' and researchers' agendas can both be met. Participants may have expectations of the researchers that cannot be fulfilled. In the work on street children, for instance, participants often asked if medical examinations would be carried out, something the research team could not provide.

Focus groups

Until the 1970s, focus groups were largely a tool of market research, where they have been used to assess consumers' views of new products and publicity. In health research, they began to be used for similar purposes in evaluating health interventions, such as family-planning programmes. Basch (1987) suggests that their adoption by health education as a useful research tool relied on both the market research tradition and the history of group processes used in health education itself as a tool for behaviour change. Focus groups are now widely used (perhaps over-used) in a range of health research and evaluation settings. In essence, a focus group is a small (usually 6–12 people) group brought together to discuss a particular issue (such as local health services, or a particular health promotion campaign) under the direction of a facilitator, who has a list of topics to discuss. Typically groups last between one and two hours and include a mixed group of participants from different social backgrounds who do not know each other. Each participant may also complete individual questionnaires to gather socio-demographic information and perhaps provide comparisons of what is said in public and private. These techniques are useful in social marketing, for instance in evaluating the suitability of health promotion materials for their intended audiences. They have also been widely used in studies looking at people's perceptions of health risks (Desvouges and Smith 1988). Focus groups have the potential for producing considerable information in a fairly short space of time on, for instance, how media messages are understood and talked about.

Natural groups

Participants in the traditional focus group have not met before the discussion. However, in social research, rather than market research, the aim is often to access *how* social knowledge about a particular topic is generated, as well as what the content of that knowledge is. To achieve this, it is often useful to use 'natural groups' or groups of people who know each other already. This maximizes interaction between participants, as well as between the facilitator and participants, and potentially provides the researcher with some access to shared group culture. Natural groups can be informal or formal. Informal groups are those that occur fortuitously in the course of fieldwork – interviews with groups of workmates, for instance, or women gathered around a new mother, as in Case Study 5.1.

Household interviews are one kind of natural group that can be a useful source of information, as the household may be a key level of social organization that impacts on health. Interviewing all the members of a household together provides access to how household-level decisions may be made. These might include decisions about access to health care, or purchasing health-related goods and services. Household interviews have been perhaps under-used in developed country settings. In informal interviews, especially if opportunistic, there will not usually be a structured topic guide, and data will be recorded through field notes rather than tape recordings. Khan and Manderson (1992) suggest that in practice, many interviews in developing country settings will be informal group interviews: as researchers start asking questions, more people will join in, and formal protocols are adapted in practice, as the everyday demands of people coming and going or work being done interrupt a focused series of questions. As they note, this can be a real bonus, as such 'natural clusterings represent ... the resources upon which any of the group might draw ... a group that may weave or repair nets together [also] provides the scripting for the management of an illness event'. The informal discussion groups formed either by design or opportunistically during fieldwork are exactly those in which health care decisions are typically made in everyday life.

Formal natural group interviews are those in which the group is invited to attend for the purposes of research. Usually, the researcher will book a private room and ask all participants to come for a specified time, and the discussion will be taped. Case Studies 5.1 and 5.2 both used natural groups for data collection. In the first, on Bedouin views of maternal child health services (Beckerleg et al. 1997), participants were interviewed in an informal setting, that of the homes of new mothers. The second, on understandings of HIV/AIDS, used more formal settings.

Advantages of using group interviews

In recent years, various kinds of group interviews have become popular in health research to offset some of the disadvantages of one-to-one interviews. In a group interview, the researcher ideally has access to interaction between the participants, as well as between the interviewer and interviewed. This, in theory, provides a more 'naturalistic' setting, resembling in some ways the kinds of interaction people might have in their everyday lives. In terms of the discussion in Chapter 2 on research designs, the focus group can therefore be used in more observational designs. In health research this is a real advantage

Case Study 5.1   Using natural groups to gather Bedouin views of maternal and child health services

(Source: Beckerleg, S., Lewando-Hundt, G.A., Borkan, J.M., Abu Saad, K.J. and Belmaker, I. (1997) 'Eliciting local voices using natural group interviews', *Anthropology and Medicine*, 4: 273–88)

Bedouin Arabs are a minority group of Israeli citizens, in socially disadvantaged circumstances. Although traditionally semi-nomadic, in recent years those living in Israel have largely been settled in towns, with many on low incomes and in poor housing conditions. Maternal and child health services are provided, for a fee, at clinics run by the Ministry of Health. As part of a larger study to improve maternal and child health care, this study aimed to consult with service users and non-users on the value and quality of the health clinics.

Previous research on child health had used structured questionnaires in home interviews with mothers. Susan Beckerleg and colleagues suggest that this approach may have been inappropriate in this cultural setting, as it is difficult to interview mothers on their own: if strangers come to the house, neighbours and family will gather to protect the mother and participate in the visit. Suspicion of outsiders might lead to inhibited discussion. Instead of attempting to interview mothers on their own, the researchers decided to talk to both women and men in groups with which they were familiar, and in which they could freely express opinions. Natural groups of men and women who would interact in everyday life were chosen to elicit views. In this setting, the most appropriate groups were family-based. To talk to women, the researchers invited women giving birth in local hospitals to take part in the study and consent to a group interview in their home during the 40-day post-partum period. Traditionally women are secluded during this time, and are visited by related women who come to drink tea and eat lunch. These visitors form an ideal natural group for interviews about maternal and child health services, as this is a time when women would talk to each other about family news and childbirth experiences. Each extended family or sub-tribe has a guest house in which men regularly meet to enjoy conversation, tea or coffee and entertain guests. To include men's views, the researchers included groups in these guest houses. The research team recruited and trained Arab Israelis to conduct and record the group interviews in pairs, matched with the participants for gender. Key issues for the participants were confidentiality and full understanding of the aims of the study. As tape recorders inhibited open discussion, data were collected through detailed notes of the discussion. These notes were translated into English if necessary before analysis.

The findings suggested that preventative health services were important to both men and women in this community, but that several barriers to use existed, including financial barriers, distance to the clinics and problems in staff–patient interaction that resulted from cultural and linguistic differences between Bedouin users and nurses from other cultures. The methods of data collection worked well for the topic of maternal and child health, which was not one of a particularly sensitive or personal nature. For more private issues (such as family planning and household finances) the researchers identified women who could be interviewed in a private setting.

when we want to access not just how people talk to each other about health matters, but also how knowledge about health is produced and reproduced in 'natural' social situations. It can also be an advantage when researching workers in health service settings. For instance, interviewing ward staff in a group allows the researcher not just to observe who says what, but also who speaks most, which kinds of staff dominate, and whose comments are taken seriously. Case Study 5.2, from research by Jenny Kitzinger and colleagues on the effect of media messages about AIDS in the UK, illustrates how the interaction between participants was as important a part of the data as the content of what was said.

A further advantage is that some sensitive issues may be more readily discussed within group settings. One example is perhaps dissatisfaction with service provision. In a one-to-one interview, it may be more difficult for interviewees to disclose negative views (especially if the interviewer is a service provider), whereas in a meeting with other service users, it can be less threatening for participants if such views come from the group, rather than from one dissatisfied individual. Helen Schneider and Natasha Palmer (2002) have a good example from this from a study of users' views of primary health care services in South Africa. They used both exit interviews (with users as they left the primary care facility) and focus groups in a study of views of service provision at 19 sites across South Africa. Although in exit interviews users were generally satisfied with the services received, in focus groups many areas of dissatisfaction were discussed, including complaints about lack of privacy, rushed consultations, and dissatisfaction with communication and treatments prescribed. Schneider and Palmer note that the focus group data are not necessarily more valid as a report of reality (indeed their transcripts contained many stories clearly told for dramatic effect, such as accounts of people dying through lack of care in the waiting rooms), but that the format does generate particular accounts that are not generated through interviews.

Clearly the kind of information that is easier to disclose in a group setting will depend on local cultural values, and the nature of the group. Asking for personal information in a 'natural' group that exists outside the research setting may not only be unproductive, but potentially unethical if the likely impact of disclosures on participants' everyday lives is not considered (see Case Study 3.1). This requires considerable sensitivity and local knowledge on the part of the research team. In their report of a study of young women's understanding of HIV transmission and their needs for AIDS prevention information in Zimbabwe, Davison Munodawafa and colleagues (1995) note the uneasiness of many of the groups in discussing their views of sexual behaviour and cultural norms. The groups they recruited were all 'natural'

Case Study 5.2   Using focus groups to study the effects of media messages about AIDS

(Sources: Kitzinger, J. (1994) 'The methodology of focus groups: the importance of interaction between the research participants', *Sociology of Health and Illness*, 16: 103–21, and Kitzinger, J. (1990) 'Audience understandings of AIDS messages: a discussion of methods', *Sociology of Health and Illness*, 12: 319–35)

The AIDS Media Research Project studied the production, content and effect of media messages about AIDS in the UK. The researchers used group interviews to examine the effects of 'how media messages are processed by audiences and how understandings of AIDS are constructed' (Kitzinger 1994: 104). Focus group discussions were chosen for their potential to provide access not just to the content of people's views, but also how those views were used and developed in everyday social interaction. For potentially sensitive subjects such as HIV/AIDS, the group setting may also encourage open discussion. The group participants were chosen to cover a wide range of different populations in the UK, including those who might be expected to have particular perspectives on the issue of AIDS. They were 'natural groups' in that they pre-existed the research, such as a group of women whose children went to the same playgroup, male workers on a gay helpline, a lesbian friendship group, a team of civil engineers who worked together, and members of a retirement club. That they were natural groups was important, as family, social and work settings are the ones in which we come to know about issues such as AIDS, and in which we develop our views. The intention was to maximize the interaction between participants in the groups to see how social knowledge was developed. As the participants knew each other already, there was also potential for access to what they did, as well as what they said they did, as other group members commented on how beliefs coexisted with everyday life. For these reasons, Kitzinger suggests that their use of natural groups is more 'naturalistic' than most research interview situations, but that it is of course an artificial research setting, in which the explicit aim is to explore often unarticulated views. Using natural groups 'allows for the collection of information both on group norms and the ways in which groups may mediate (relay, censor, selectively highlight and oppose) media messages' (Kitzinger 1990: 321).

To maximize interaction, facilitators used a number of techniques. First, group exercises allowed the participants to warm up and start to discuss the issues with physical prompts. These included cards with statements about who was 'at risk' from AIDS, which participants had to sort into groups of differing risk levels. This encouraged group participants to talk to each other, and to verbalize their reasoning. Another exercise was the 'News Game' in which the group was split into two teams, given a set of pictures and asked to construct a news report about AIDS. The pictures were taken from television news and documentary reports. The final exercise involved a health promotion advert from which the slogan ('How to recognize someone with HIV') had been removed. Participants were asked whether they recalled any adverts about HIV/AIDS, then asked to speculate on what the slogan was. Finally, the slogan was revealed and participants were asked to comment on the actual slogan and other parts of the text.

The second method for encouraging interaction was the use of the facilitator's skills in actively managing the discussion, pushing participants into accounting for their views, or exploring disagreements. Maximizing interaction allowed the researchers access not only to what people thought, but also to the cultural contexts in which views were held. Thus jokes, and the levels of agreement and disagreements between participants, suggested group norms, and the ways in which certain views are legitimate or not in the social settings in which they live and work. Even natural groups are not homogeneous, though, and Kitzinger notes the ways in which group participants were often surprised by differences in opinions amongst them. Disagreements forced participants to account for the views they held, and gave the researchers a chance to see what arguments are convincing in everyday interaction.

The exercises such as the card game were also useful sources of data on the assumptions participants made, where their knowledge came from, and for identifying areas of confusion and misinformation. The cards had descriptions of types of people taken from an opinion survey of the public, including 'people who donate blood at a blood donor centre'. In the discussion about how at risk this group was, it became clear that many participants assumed that the description referred to those who received donated blood, rather than the donors. This provides real insight into the meaning of survey results that suggest the public misunderstand risk activities. Participants' interpretations of the health education advert were also illuminating for showing how such images can be read in quite different ways from those intended by health educators. The advert was intended to persuade readers that there was no way of telling by looking at people whether they were HIV-positive or not – that they looked exactly like other people. In a minority of groups, participants read the image as meaning that there was a distinctive 'look' of someone who was HIV-positive or had AIDS.

groups of women aged 15 to 22 who would work and socialize together after the research had finished, including self-help groups organized through local mining company and church organizations. The research team used several methods to reduce the potential for embarrassment. First, they reassured the young women that men would not be allowed to come to the discussion, or to listen at a distance. They also assured them of confidentiality, by ensuring that no participant identified themselves or others by name during the session. Young female group moderators were recruited, who were not only fluent in the local languages, but also at ease talking with other women about AIDS and sexual issues. Group discussions were held in a relaxed atmosphere, with refreshments and dancing before and after the focus group. Finally, the disclosure of sensitive personal information during the discussion was discouraged by the moderator.

What is and is not sensitive information is of course culturally specific. A discussion of knowledge about condoms, HIV risk and AIDS may be sensitive for young women in Zimbabwe, but not older women in London, whereas the latter might feel that a discussion of household income was too 'private' for a focus group.

Naturalism

The methodological strength of group interviews is that they supposedly approximate a more 'natural' interaction than individual interviews, thus providing the researcher with access to how people talk to each other about particular topics. The implication is that the researcher will capture some of the advantages of ethnographic research (see Chapter 6) in a focused way without the time-consuming and arduous business of actually carrying out fieldwork. A well-facilitated group has the feel of an everyday discussion, with participants interacting, joking and arguing with each other, rather than through the facilitator. However, it should be remembered that any specifically gathered or facilitated group is not a 'natural' setting, and that there are few situations in everyday life when peers come together to discuss one topic for a lengthy period of time, and few in which they are conscious of their utterances being treated as 'data'. In most group interviews, a facilitator also 'controls' the interaction to a greater or lesser extent, by deliberately canvassing views, controlling turn-taking or asking for elaboration from participants. This facilitation obviously shapes to a greater or lesser extent the accounts participants give, and what they consider to be relevant to the researcher's needs.

It also has to be remembered that, for participants, the discussion itself is of course another source of both information and beliefs, in that it is one forum in which participants *come to know* particular things. The experience of taking part in a group interview may clarify, elaborate and even change participants' views. The following extract is taken from a study of how people with glaucoma cope with symptoms (Green et al. 2002b), and is part of a long exchange in which participants trade stories about the everyday difficulties caused by their eyesight problems. It is clear that taking part in the focus group has started to change the way in which one respondent (R4) thinks about her difficulties, with her beginning to see the possibility of them being 'symptoms' rather than just problems of daily living:

R1: I can't follow things – and even, I go to church and, we've got large print hymn books and they are large print, you know – I can't even carry them!
R2: I have the same problem! And there's another problem . . . putting your underwear on . . . underslips you know, they have a seam down the side – I have to feel for the seam, otherwise often I come out with my underslip on inside out.

R3: Mm
R1: Oh yes!
R4: ... I'm wondering, listening to you, because I have a job to recognize textures ... so maybe it's the glaucoma that does that.

In terms of generating more data about the impact of glaucoma on everyday life, the interaction in this group was an advantage, as other people's stories prompted group members both to remember, and to frame as significant, their own experiences. But the research setting itself has generated these data: there are clearly 'experiences of glaucoma' that are only recognized as such once other people help to frame them in this way. Similarly, in a focus group study of consumers' views of food safety, several participants mentioned during the discussion that taking part had made them think more about food safety, or that they had learnt about risks they hadn't known about beforehand from other participants (Green et al. 2003). The group interview does not just, then, 'collect' pre-existing ideas and viewpoints, but can be part of the process by which these views are produced. Whether this constitutes a methodological problem or not depends on the aim of the study. If groups are used as part of a participatory design, in which developing the participants' understanding of a particular issue may be an explicit aim, it is clearly an advantage. It is also an advantage if research aims are to explore this process of knowledge production, rather than merely document the views of participants. For more positivist studies, in which group interviews are used as a tool for a survey of participants' views, this can look like 'contamination': the data produced reflect the opinions or beliefs that people develop during the process of the group discussion itself, rather than any pre-existing beliefs or opinions that they might have outside the research setting.

At a practical level, one disadvantage is that the more 'natural' a group discussion is, the harder it may be to analyse as data. The following extract comes from a focus group discussion with children from a study of children's views of accident risks. The participants were classmates who lived near each other in the same housing, which consisted of high-rise blocks of flats. The discussion was 'successful' in that there was considerable interaction between the children, who interrupted and spoke over each other in their eagerness to contribute, as can be seen in the passage transcribed here. The extract follows the children listing risks for fire in their homes, and concerns a debate about what would happen in the event of a fire in the flats:

R1: Would you jump out of the window or get burnt to pieces?
R2: I'd jump out of the window
R1: But if you lived on the fourth floor you'd be scared –
R3: If you lived on the top floor . . . and your house is on fire . . . how you gonna get out? You can't jump out of the window because you'd be dead!
R4: If you –
R1: No, listen, if you could jump from the balcony –
? You'd go splat on the floor and die

? – no, you wouldn't die –
? – you will die –
? – jump carefully –
? – you could land on your feet –
? – your legs would break –
? – how would your legs break?
R1: – if your legs would break just like that, you wouldn't be able to walk for the rest of your life (Green and Hart 1999: 25)

Although this provides rich access to the kinds of discussion children might have without a facilitator present, it is perhaps limited as data, beyond telling us about the kinds of 'accident stories' that will be told spontaneously. The audio-tape of this section of the discussion was almost impossible to transcribe, as the number of unidentified speakers testifies, and as the participants all speak at once it is difficult to separate out particular points of view or how they are utilized in persuading others.

In other discussion groups held as part of this study of children's views of accidents, the young people themselves 'policed' the discussion to some extent, especially when the groups were held on school premises. In these more formal settings, children are used to calmer discussions, in which teachers or other adults will tightly control turn-taking so that only one child speaks at once, and everyone has a turn. When facilitating groups in school settings, we noticed that children would raise their hand before making a point, or insist that their peers took turns in speaking. In non-school settings, such as youth clubs, the discussions were less structured and there was more interaction between the children themselves (Green and Hart 1999). This illustrates the contextual nature of focus group data. Participants take on an appropriate social role, which is to some extent determined by the setting, and their contributions reflect this. What is appropriate to say in a youth club may not be appropriate to say in a school, even if away from the classroom and teachers. In other settings, of course, these contexts may have very different meanings. Baker and Hinton (1999), whose work in Nepal was referred to above, discuss the particular context of research with people living in refugee camps. Here, in contrast to the UK-based study, schools were a preferred location, as the researchers were seen as providers of services or material aid in other settings. Similarly, they argue that the home (with its lack of privacy) may be a less desirable setting than a relatively public space. The key point is that data from group interviews, like any other data, must be analysed with regard to the context in which they are produced, and the local meanings of that context. Care must be taken not merely to take particular utterances by individual participants as reified 'opinions' or 'views' without situating them within these structures of production.

Wilkinson and Kitzinger (2000) discuss a useful example of this in their work on the value of 'feeling positive' in studies of people with cancer. They suggest that much of the research that underpins the concept of 'feeling positive' is flawed because it takes little account of the ways in which people talk about 'feeling positive' in everyday settings. Using examples from their focus group study of women with breast cancer they show how, when participants talk about 'feeling positive', it would be a mistake to read this off as merely indicating some underlying mental state. Instead, they point to the ways in which the term is actually used interactively in the focus group talk. First, it is used as an idiom – an ordinary saying that is used in a formulaic way to summarize 'what everyone thinks' and to keep a conversation moving along. Phrases such as 'you've got to think positive' are ways of generating agreement in general in discussions. They are difficult to disagree with, and may be used at points where the speaker is seeking support and affirmation from others. Second, they note that if particular attention is paid to what participants are 'thinking positively' about, it is clear that it is not having cancer, but about other things in life or the possibility of recovery. Third, comments about 'thinking positive' are often made just after participants speak about difficult issues, such as feeling devastated by the diagnosis. The comment is thus used conversationally to enable participants to discuss emotional or difficult issues, which would be difficult to do in a group unless followed by a routine positive comment.

This kind of analysis clearly relies on cultural as well as linguistic knowledge to understand the ways in which particular phrases are used interactively, as well as what the content of them might mean. The issue of language was discussed in detail in Chapter 4, and the same principles apply to group interview data, which also requires some attention to the *ways* in which talk is used in particular settings.

Limitations

The advantages of group interviews are also their limitations. Group settings may be ideal for accessing cultural norms, and how they are reproduced in everyday talk, but this means they are perhaps less useful for accessing in–depth accounts of socially deviant or marginal opinions. Group dynamics, with the dominance of particular group members, are a useful indicator of the hierarchy of opinions, and the ways in which marginal ones are 'silenced', but of course also limit the expression or elaboration of less acceptable opinions or the views of those lower in a status hierarchy. Thus, using ward-based natural groups to look at the views of health professionals in a hospital may be a useful way of accessing how various professionals talk to each other, but the more junior staff may feel too inhibited to speak out, or to disagree with senior staff. Again, the aims of the study will determine how far this is a problem. In the study on children's views of accident risks, referred to above, the aim was to capture how peer groups of young people interpret accident prevention messages and provide some useful information for planning health promotion materials for this age group. In many of the group discussions, young people discussed peers who were perceived as 'accident-prone' in derogatory terms. These children were to some extent stigmatized for their clumsiness. If we had wanted to look at the experiences of these children specifically, the dynamics of a focus group would have been inappropriate – the most 'accident-prone' children would have been unlikely to speak about their views within this dominant culture. Marginal or less socially acceptable views are unlikely to be explored in a group setting and may be best accessed in the more private setting of a one-to-one interview.

Local cultural and political considerations can also limit the range of views expressed in community interviews. Coreil (1995) discusses her experience of using community interviews in a participatory project designed to evaluate community management of a water system in Rwanda. Participants were recruited from users of standpipes in the locality, and although attendance at the meetings was good, with most turning into large community gatherings, women were under-represented. Not only did women have domestic responsibilities, which limited the time they had available to attend meetings, but also they traditionally had less involvement with public meetings. Those who did come did not speak much. 'Community interviews' may only access the views of particular (higher status) groups in the community, and in many settings may marginalize women's voices or the socially excluded.

Practical issues

The kind of group interview needed for the research will, then, depend on what kind of data you are aiming to produce. A focus group may well be appropriate for research that aims to gather a broad range of responses to, say, a proposed health promotion campaign, whereas interviews with less formal natural groups may be preferred if the aim is to gather more naturalistic data on how knowledge about a health topic is formed in social interaction. For any kind of organized group interview (as opposed to opportunistic ones carried out in the course of fieldwork), the practicalities of organizing group interviews need considering quite carefully for the method to work well. This will involve planning how participants will be sampled and recruited, what the topic guide will include (including ice-breaking and focusing prompts), how the groups will be run, where you will hold them, and how data will be recorded.

Sampling

The previous chapter outlined some of the principles of sampling participants for interviews, and the same principles apply to focus groups. Essentially the aim of a sampling strategy is to maximize the opportunity of producing enough data to answer the research question. How this is achieved will depend on the research question, feasibility, resources and the setting. Convenience samples, based on networks of contacts, may be sufficient for exploratory or pilot studies. More systematic purposive sampling strategies will be needed for most studies in order to generate representative data that will be credible to users. One common strategy is to identify, from the literature and pilot work, the key demographic variables that are likely to have an impact on participants' views of the topic. These then form a 'sampling grid', and groups can be recruited to reflect various combinations of variables. To take an example, in a European study of consumers' attitudes to the risk of BSE and other food risks (Draper et al. 2002), 'point in the life-cycle' was identified from the literature as a key influence on attitudes to food risk. Four important life-cycle groups were selected: adolescents, who are primarily reliant on others for choosing their food; 'young singles', who are responsible for their own food; 'family food purchasers', who choose food for their children as well as themselves; and 'older citizens', who may have memories of war-time food-rationing. In addition, in the UK it was known that geographical locality (whether urban and rural) and income (whether low income or more affluent) were likely to have an impact on attitudes to risk. Three other countries were involved in the study (Finland, Germany and Italy) and researchers there followed the same life-cycle segments and chose appropriate variables relevant to their own populations and what was known about differences in consumer behaviour. In Italy, for instance, the key difference was region, with sites selected in the north and south of the country. In the UK, eleven groups were selected to cover these key demographic differences (see Box 5.2).

The intention is to both represent the range of groups likely to have a different orientation to the topic, and also provide some comparative data. Thus, the different life-cycle groups can be compared with each other, or with the different income groups. Using the same life-cycle groups in four countries also meant we could compare the views of, for instance, family food purchasers or older citizens cross-nationally. There are limits to using the same

---

Box 5.2   Sampling grid for UK groups in study of public perceptions of BSE risk in Europe

	Adolescents	Singles	Family food purchasers	Older citizens
Low income:				
rural	×		×	
urban	×	×	×	×
Affluent:				
rural			×	×
urban	×	×	×	

× = one group.

Source: Draper et al. (2002).

sampling frame in cross-national studies, as clearly demographic variables have different meanings in different settings. The groups of adolescents worked well in the UK study, as young people (aged 14 to 16) were already making some decisions about food choices, but less well in Italy where they reported merely that their mothers were the primary decision-makers, and they had little to say on the issue. This sampling strategy also becomes unwieldy with a large number of population segments. Adding in, for instance, gender or ethnicity would have led to a very large number of cells.

Recruitment

Recruiting participants can be time-consuming, and frustrating if attendance is poor. Many researchers have had the experience of booking rooms and sending reminders only to have few or no participants attending. Clearly the likely level of non-attendance will depend on how involved the researchers are with the participants' community, the interest of the community in the research topic, and the perceived benefits and gains of attending a group discussion. It is usually advisable to over-recruit by about 25 per cent, thus inviting 15 people if you are aiming to include 12 in the discussion, but in some settings higher over-recruitment will be needed. In other settings, of course, where it might be common to bring kin and neighbours, over-recruitment may be a problem, in which case some provision needs to be made to entertain 'extras' if there are too many participants arriving.

-- Once it has been decided which groups will be sampled, there are three potential strategies for recruiting participants. The first, and probably least satisfactory, is opportunism. To recruit 'natural' groups, key 'gatekeepers' or contacts are invited to recruit their peers. Networks of personal contacts can be good gatekeepers for workplace and social groups, especially for pilot or exploratory studies. Nevertheless, however extensive the personal networks of the research team are, they are unlikely to generate a representative sample or to include all the population segments of interest. Advertising is one possibility, although most experience suggests it does not work well. Identifying community groups to work with is more productive. Community leaders can be asked to help contact key people to invite them. This may be the only way of including 'hard to reach' population groups. In a study of bilingual children's views of their experiences of interpreting for family members in health service settings, we contacted cultural centres, after-school activity groups and language schools to recruit bilingual young people. One disadvantage of working with established community groups is that it can be difficult to determine the sampling, and the researcher is reliant on community leaders to identify appropriate people to contact.

The second strategy is systematically inviting people, either as individuals, or as contacts for their peer groups, from a sampling frame, if there is one, for the population of interest. Such a sampling frame might be, for example, a list of all patients at a particular clinic, all nursing students in a college or all mothers giving birth in hospital (as in the example in Case Study 5.1). A sample of participants can then be drawn randomly from this list, or more purposively if you are aiming for a particular mix in each group. Unless the topic is of great interest to participants, this method may have low response rates. Using incentives, such as payments, refreshments or vouchers, can increase participation.

Third, commercial market research companies are one possibility for recruiting particular groups in short time scales and for groups that might be 'hard to reach'. Most have large databases of potential participants, and can recruit the required number of people in each demographic group needed fairly quickly. They are of course relatively expensive, and pay higher fees to participants than is usual in social research. The groups constituted have other drawbacks. The main one is that participants can be, to some extent, professional 'focus groupees', who may be adept at adopting particular social roles for the purposes of research discussions. This may not matter, and indeed raises a question about how far the focus groups we recruit are adopting particular positions on the basis of how they were recruited. Most of us have a range of social roles (work-based, family-based, interest-based) and gathering a group of 'East African women with HIV' or 'elderly men with diabetes' to discuss issues of service use does presuppose that these identities shape the kinds of knowledge displayed.

Incentives

Following the example of market research companies, it can sometimes be beneficial to offer some incentive to participate, particularly for focus groups, in which the participant's stake in the research may be less than in more participatory studies. Incentives might include reimbursing travel and child care expenses, providing refreshments, or offering some kind of payment, or payment in kind, such as store vouchers. Offering incentives is more common than in one-to-one interview research simply because the researcher is often asking more of the group participant: they have to attend at a set time and place, rather than one convenient for them, the time taken is often more burdensome, and out-of-pocket expenses such as child care and transport are needed. In countries with a tradition of market research, participants may well expect some kind of small payment, unless the study is one closely tied to their own interests. However, in academic health research the use of incentives is often rather contentious, with suggestions that we may be 'biasing' response, and they may not be appropriate (or possible) in all settings.

The topic guide

A topic guide is a more or less structured interview schedule for the discussion, consisting of a small number of questions, with follow-up prompts to use to generate further discussion. The early prompts should be general, moving on to more specific issues. Box 5.3 shows the topic guide for the study of European consumers' attitudes to food risk, focusing on their views of BSE.

Box 5.3   Protocol for a focus group discussion

Public perceptions of BSE in Europe

Protocol for focus group discussions

Groups to last 1–2 hours.

Group Task 1 (15 minutes):
'Order the following foods from the ones you feel most confident are safe to
    eat, to the ones you feel least confident are safe to eat'
Large cards with following words/pictures: Meat, Poultry, Fish, Eggs, Dairy
    Produce, Fruit & Vegetables

Group Task 2 (15 minutes):
'One food concern is BSE [check everyone has heard of this] – please sort
    the following foods in terms of how much of a risk you think they have of
    being contaminated with BSE'
Large cards with following words/pictures: Beef Steak, Ox Tail, Minced Meat,
    Dairy Foods

Prompts for general discussion (50 minutes):
1   Generally, do you think the food available is safe to eat?
2   Is it as safe as it used to be?
3   Whose responsibility is it to make food safe?
4   Who do you trust for information on food safety?
5   Do you worry about BSE? (Why? Why not?)
6   Why do you think BSE has happened?
7   Have you changed your/your family's consumption of beef because of
    BSE? (If so, what has replaced it?)

Conclusion/Debrief (5 minutes):
Ask each participant in turn if there is anything they want to add. Thank
participants, ask them to complete brief questionnaire, hand out travel
expenses and ask if they have further questions about the study.

Source: Adapted from Draper et al. (2002).

Ice-breaking tasks and focusing exercises

Ice-breaking exercises are primarily designed to generate discussion between
the participants early on, so that everyone has a chance to speak and get to
know each other enough to interact. Even when using natural groups, where
people already know each other, an introductory exercise can establish preferred titles (whether participants want to use first names, or last names, or
pseudonyms) and individual voices, so they can be identified on the tape.
Focusing exercises are designed to get the group to orient themselves to the
topic in hand, and sometimes to gather particular kinds of data. Case Study 5.2
has some examples of exercises used to explore how media messages about

AIDS are interpreted and framed by groups, and the protocol for the European BSE study in Box 5.3 has examples of two group tasks. These examples are both exercises designed to generate data through facilitating members of the group talking to each other about the topic. The study by Munodawafa and colleagues (1995) on young women's understanding of HIV transmission in Zimbabwe, referred to above, used dancing to relax participants before the discussion. Ice-breaking activities need choosing with care. Not everyone feels comfortable with these kinds of 'games' and for some participants the embarrassment of joining in can cause considerable discomfort. Tasks requiring cards to be read are clearly unsuitable for participants with limited literacy skills, and pictures or physical props can be used instead.

Running a group

The role of the facilitator (sometimes called a 'moderator' in focus group studies) is vital. Like any interviewer, their job is to establish a relaxed atmosphere, enable participants to tell their stories, and listen actively. This involves greeting participants as they arrive, handing out refreshments, information sheets and consent forms if necessary, introducing any ice-breaking tasks and prompting each new topic. This is too much work for one person, and most groups are run by a facilitator plus a note-taker, or assistant. The second person keeps written notes and ensures that tape recorders are working and switched on. If notes are the only form of data collected, they can also summarize at key points for the group, to check that views are being recorded reliably.

The skills needed to facilitate a discussion are similar to those needed for any interviewing, i.e. the ability to listen actively, be non-judgemental, and encourage others to speak (by not interrupting, adopting relaxed body language, making right visual and verbal cues, not jumping in too quickly with the next question or prompt). Facilitators do not have to be an expert on the topic – in fact it is usually helpful if they are not, so that participants are not inhibited in discussing their views.

How far the facilitator actively manages the discussion depends on the aim of the group, and how tightly structured the topic guide is. If each group needs to cover all the topics on the guide, the facilitator will need to be careful to move the discussion on if it deviates too much from the guide. In more exploratory work, the 'deviations' can be left to run for a little longer, as topics that seem irrelevant at the time may be crucial at the analysis stage for making sense of people's understanding.

Setting

The physical setting is important. Ideally this should be a quiet, comfortable room where there will be no disturbances, although some trade-off may be necessary between accessibility and suitability for research purposes. A local community centre room may be less quiet, but more accessible and familiar and less intimidating to the group than a university or hospital seminar room.

Recording data

Ideally, two good-quality tape recorders are needed to record a group discussion, in addition to a note-taker. In rural developing country settings tape recording may be impossible, or inappropriate. In this case, it is useful to summarize the views of the group as the discussion progresses, so that the facilitator can check they have understood the key points. In literate communities, these summaries can be written on large sheets of paper throughout the discussion.

Sensitive issues

Great care must be taken in running discussions on sensitive topics, especially with natural groups who have to live, work or socialize together after the researchers have gone home. A good facilitator is likely to be skilled in getting participants to feel safe, and to reveal stories that they might not have shared in everyday settings, but this of course raises issues about how far the researchers need to protect participants from over-disclosure (see Case Study 3.1). However bland or non-controversial the topic appears to be, taking part in a group discussion may raise sensitive issues for some members of the group. As Michael Bloor and colleagues note in their book on focus groups (Bloor et al. 2001: 55–6), the research interview is not a therapeutic group, and if participants do get upset, or make disclosures that may be difficult for them later, researchers should not attempt to engage in 'therapy', but debrief quietly at the end of the session. For particularly sensitive topics, it is worth finding out the telephone numbers of appropriate service providers in case participants do ask for further help. Participants may also raise issues that are difficult for facilitators, if they express strong emotions or extreme views that are not those of the facilitator. In the research described in Case Study 5.2, Kitzinger reports some extreme homophobic views from some groups. On issues likely to generate this kind of data, it may be sensible to ensure that there is also scope for the facilitator to 'debrief' after the group. A formal arrangement with a trusted colleague or supervisor may be needed for the facilitator to talk through the experiences of conducting the group interview and their feelings and reactions to it.

Developing appropriate methods for the setting

The key to running successful group interviews is to ensure that the methods used are appropriate for the setting, topic and participants. If working in unfamiliar settings, it is essential to work with partners who are sensitive to cultural norms about interaction, and what will be appropriate in terms of facilitation and structure. Bilkis Vissandjée and colleagues (2002) report their experiences of running focus groups in rural Gujarat in India, in which extensive local collaboration was necessary to develop appropriate protocols. The ethical implications of this were described in Case Study 3.1. Other issues they had to take into account included: when and what to offer in the way of refreshments, what characteristics the moderator would need, and how to introduce a tape recorder to groups who may be suspicious of being recorded. As described in Case Study 3.1, the rural setting had a number of implications for ethical methodology, including ensuring confidentiality, given that in small village communities the participants are well known to each other, and complex social relationships patterned what could be said in particular settings. Thus, whether groups included mothers-in-law or village elders had considerable impact on what women could say, and the researchers supplemented the group discussions with some individual interviews. In summary, they suggest a number of rules of thumb for what they call culturally competent focus groups: flexibility, taking time to understand local customs, consulting others with research experience in the area, engaging local communities in the research design, and being prepared to adapt protocols to make use of culturally appropriate techniques of data collection. Although Vissandjée and colleagues are reflecting on their experience in rural India, these rules of thumb are useful reminders for designing appropriate group interviews in all settings.

Conclusion

Group interviews are a flexible method for producing data on social interaction, and their key advantage is that they provide access to how people display, use and construct their social knowledge as well as access to what the content of that knowledge is. In this chapter we have concentrated on two kinds of group interview commonly used in health research, the focus group (with its traditions in market research) and the 'natural' group, which attempts to recreate naturalistic social interaction in a research setting. The key to using group interviews is to remember that, as with other methods of producing data, the researcher must be aware of the context of the data production, and account for how the particular setting produced data on views, or experiences, or beliefs. Utterances made in group interview transcripts cannot be stripped of their context and presented as the essential 'views' of the participants.

KEY POINTS

- Group interviews have the key advantage of providing access to social inter-action, and thus the process of how knowledge is acquired, shared and contested in quasi-naturalistic settings.
- However, it must be remembered that group interviews are not 'natural' set-tings, and the context of data collection must be taken into account in the analysis.
- The protocol for running a group discussion has to be appropriate for the setting and population.

EXERCISE

Consider any professional or local community with which you are familiar. Design a protocol for a study using 'natural' groups from this community on one of the following topics:

1 Barriers to giving up smoking.
2 Dealing with stress at work.
3 Using dental services.

Include in your protocol appropriate ice-breaking and focusing exercises and some prompts to facilitate the discussion. What particular issues would working on this topic with this community raise in terms of: confiden-tiality, the impact of the research on participants after the group discussions had finished, sensitive issues, identifying an appropriate facilitator, recruit-ment?

FURTHER READING

Krueger, R. and Casey, M.A. (2000) *Focus groups: a practical guide for applied research* (3rd ed.). Thousand Oaks, CA: Sage. A useful guidebook orientated towards the practical issues of planning, recruiting, running, analysing and reporting focus groups. The authors draw from their own experiences of running different kinds of focus groups, largely in North America.

Barbour, R. and Kitzinger, J. (eds) (1999) *Developing focus group research: politics, theory and practice.* London: Sage. A collection of chapters draw-ing on authors' empirical experiences of focus group research that cover methodological issues including the impact of context, using focus groups in feminist and participatory research, using focus groups for sensitive topics, and approaches to analysis.

Bloor, M., Frankland, J., Thomas, M. and Robson, K. (2001) *Focus groups in social research.* London: Sage. Discusses the contribution of focus group methods to social research, including a chapter on the develop-ment of 'virtual' focus groups using e-mail and Internet technology. Good discussions of the methodological weaknesses of focus group designs for many research questions.

6

Observational Methods

CHAPTER SUMMARY

The strength of observational methods is that they provide data on phenomena (such as behaviour), as well as on people's accounts of those phenomena. They can be divided into participant methods, where the researcher is present to some extent in the field studied, and non–participant methods, where researchers observe a field without involvement, through for instance analysing audio-tapes of encounters. Ethnographic accounts using participant observation have contributed detailed knowledge of how health beliefs are embedded in culture. The practical and methodological issues raised by ethnographic research, including doing ethnography close to home, rapid appraisal methods and pseudo-patient studies, are discussed, and this chapter briefly discusses the possibilities of using non–participant methods using analysis of naturally occurring data such as recordings of consultations in medical practice.

Aims of observational methods

If the aim of research is to understand a phenomenon, rather than people's accounts of it, then observational methods are often cited as the 'gold standard' of qualitative methods, given that they provide direct access to what people do, as well as what they say they do. As Becker and Geer (1957) put it:

> The most complete form of the sociological datum ... is the form in which the parti-
> cipant observer gathers it: An observation of some social event, the events which precede
> and follow it, and explanations of its meaning by participants and spectators, before,
> during and after its occurrence. Participant observation can thus provide a yardstick
> against which to measure the completeness of data gathered in other ways, a model
> which can serve to let us know what orders of information escape us when we use
> other methods. (Becker and Geer 1957: 28)

Interviews, in this 'classic' account of the strengths of observational methods, are flawed by only providing a partial account of a phenomenon. Observational methods allow the researcher to record the mundane and unre-markable (to participants) features of everyday life that interviewees might not feel were worth commenting on and the context within which they occur. Similarly, for Lofland (1971), participant observation is a route to 'knowing people' rather than 'knowing about them'. This perspective, that observational strategies somehow allow the researchers closer to some essential truth about social life, is implicit in much qualitative social research. The 'purest' form of data is that gathered directly from naturally occurring situations, in which behaviour and responses to it can be observed in situ. The idea of observational data being the 'gold standard' in terms of their validity is also a common theme in health research, with observations often provided as illustrating the truth about some event or process, in (often ironic) contrast to interview accounts, or statistical records. Certainly, there are a number of examples of observational studies on health topics that have demonstrated very nicely the limitations of other sources of data (such as official records) in terms of their reliability or validity.

Isobel Bowler (1995), for instance, draws on her observations of a maternity hospital in southern England to show how official statistics and 'facts' about women of south Asian descent result from particular bureaucratic processes, embedded in cultural practices, such as stereotypical assumptions made by staff. These particular social practices result in flawed records about women of south Asian descent. Examples include observations of record-making when women were booked onto the ward, when Bowler observed 'facts' such as nationality being recorded in line with what staff assumed about the women in front of them, rather than their actual answers, and details of their medical histories being missed because of difficulties in using standard forms with tick box answers. Another example was date of birth – for the staff, an unremarkable 'fact' that everyone would know, but for a few patients of south Asian descent, not a significant 'fact' about themselves, but one that they had learnt to respond to by estimating the year of birth and giving 1 January as the date. Bowler's observations thus provide essential information for anyone utilizing hospital records as a source of data on maternity patients, and point to some of the ways in which such records are likely to be incomplete or incorrect.

In a similar vein, Gillian Lewando-Hundt and her colleagues (Lewando-Hundt et al. 1999) looked at official statistics about birth in the Gaza Strip. Here, observational data explained why address data was missing from registrations, and also suggested that birth weight was often recorded erroneously (see discussion in Chapter 2). The findings from the observational study, suggest Lewando-Hundt and colleagues, demonstrate the unique contribution of qualitative methods:

> [Anthropology], as well as explaining how social systems function, can make explicit the ways in which people use documentation to cope. ... Anthropology can make its contribution to epidemiology. It is precisely here that qualitative methods can be used to validate health surveillance data and guide policy intervention. (Lewando-Hundt et al. 1999: 842)

Thus observational data are widely assumed to be the archetypal qualitative method, producing the most valid data on social behaviour, and demonstrating the unique contribution qualitative methods can make to researching health. Of course, this perspective does make some rather positivist and empiricist assumptions, in which there is a rather idealistic view of the 'real', which can be reflected by a trained observer's eye, and perfectly recreated in the research write-up. It also assumes that all research questions relate to understanding phenomena directly, whereas in many cases the researcher is interested in accounts, or narratives, for which interviews are an appropriate method. However, observational methods do have methodological advantages for many health research questions, and are perhaps underused, especially in applied research, in part because of the time-consuming nature of many approaches.

Participant and non-participant observation

A classic typology of observational methods was suggested by Gold (1958), who distinguished between potential roles the researcher can adopt in terms of how much they participate in the field being observed (Figure 6.1). At one end of Gold's scale, the complete participant is a researcher who is a 'native' in the field they are observing. This includes reflexive 'insider accounts', written by professionals or patients drawing on their own experiences as data for understanding a particular issue. There is a tradition of 'sociological autobiography' in which personal experiences are used to explore theoretical or conceptual issues. Christopher Adamson (1997), for instance, draws on a detailed diary he kept

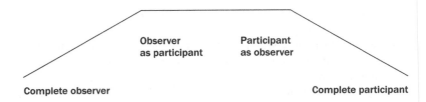

Figure 6.1   *Gold's ideal types of research role.*

while ill with and being treated for inflammatory bowel disease and his medical notes to explore how 'existential and clinical uncertainty are mutually inter-meshed properties of the medical encounter' (Adamson 1997: 138). Joel Richman (2000) used his experiences of time in intensive care as data for a paper on 'intensive care syndrome', which discussed how the environment of intensive care contributes to post-operative psychiatric disorder. In studies such as these, experiences only become 'data' in retrospect, and at the time there may be no intention to use them analytically. Less formally, many research studies begin as reflections on everyday experiences, and our own experiences as users of health services and professionals are an invaluable source of data and ideas for research questions.

However, in most studies the researcher is to some extent entering a field explicitly in order to research it. The next roles identified by Gold, the parti-cipant as observer and observer as participant roles, describe classic *ethnographic* studies, in which the researcher participates to a greater or lesser extent in the field that they are studying. Ethnography can be defined as a method of research in which the researcher 'participates, overtly or covertly, in people's daily lives for an extended period of time, watching what happens, listening to what is being said, asking questions; in fact collecting whatever data are avail-able to throw light on the issues with which he or she is concerned' (Hammersley and Atkinson 1983: 2).

When describing research methods, the term 'ethnography' is often used interchangeably with 'participant observation'. It also refers to the *product* of ethnographic investigation; that is, the written report is also called an ethno-graphy. In traditional anthropological studies, doing ethnography could entail many months or even years living in a small-scale community in order to understand the social structure and local culture. In these studies, the research design is primarily about the exposure to another culture, and the way in which the researcher comes to understand it, rather than a particular data collection method (such as 'observation'). Joseph Opala and François Boillot (1996) describe the aims of this kind of anthropology thus:

> The anthropologist can grasp a culture's world view only through long exposure. The researcher should ideally learn the language and live in the community for a year or more, spending as much time as possible interacting with people and absorbing their mode of reasoning. ... The anthropologist can also find clues through the careful observation of

art, ritual and religion where ideas normally only hinted at are often brought to the surface. (Opala and Boillot 1996: 4)

Ethnography is, then, a holistic approach to research, involving interviews, observation and the interpretation of material culture. However, the *techniques* from this kind of ethnographic work, including the observation of 'naturally occurring interaction', have been used in health research both in studying health beliefs of communities and in understanding health care organization.

Finally, at the other end of Gold's scale, the researcher can be a complete observer, and not participate in the field at all. Non-participant methods include the study of naturally occurring data, such as video-tapes of consultations in health care settings, in which the researcher is not even present in the field. They can also include studies in which the researcher is present to collect data, but does not interact with participants. This might include studies of patient behaviour in a clinic waiting room. These various roles generate rather different methodological problems. To start, we shall explore the contributions of ethnographic participant observation to health research.

Ethnography and participant observation

Classic anthropological monographs are the outcome of considerable time living with a small-scale community, coming to understand in a holistic way their beliefs and social structure, including kinship structures, religious beliefs, political systems and material culture. Medical anthropology focuses on health beliefs and healing systems. Through living and working with the community, the anthropologist comes to see the world through their eyes and understand in detail how beliefs are embedded in local cultures. The first aim of an in–depth observational study in anthropology is, then, to produce an account of a social setting that is faithful to the perspectives of the participants.

What separates this from a common–sense account of the world is that it is not *merely* an 'insider' description, but also a theoretical description. Thus an empathetic and detailed description, although perhaps intrinsically interesting, is not enough. The 'insider' view must be related to the 'outsider' view, which brings in an analytical approach to social life. This entails a sensitivity to patterns in social behaviour, and regularities that indicate underlying 'rules' of social behaviour. Anthropologists distinguish *emic* and *etic* perspectives to label these activities. The emic perspective is that of 'insiders', or the explanation of a social world provided by a participant in it. The etic perspective is that of the analyst. In his account of analysing the ritual symbols used by the Ndembu of Zambia, Victor Turner (1967) discusses the role of the anthropologist in analysing meaning as well as merely recording the participants' own interpretations:

How then, can an anthropologist justify his claim to be able to interpret a society's ritual symbols more deeply and comprehensively than the actors themselves? [F]irst . . .

he can place this ritual in its significant field setting and describe the structure and properties of that field ... the anthropologist has no particular bias and can observe the real interconnections and conflicts between groups and persons. (Turner 1967: 26–7)

The tension between an etic and an emic perspective is what drives an ethnographic analysis. It is also a tension that has practical implications, in terms of the roles adopted by the researcher engaged in any kind of participant observation. One way of describing this tension in fieldwork roles is to use the metaphors of the 'native' and the 'stranger from Mars' for potential stances the researcher can take. Thus, ideally, an ethnographer has to move between an understanding that resembles that of a 'native' participant, whether this is an urban slum dweller or an operating theatre nurse, and the complete alien, who is a naïve outsider trying to make sense of local culture: why things are done the way they are and how people account for them. The value of the 'native' perspective is that it allows an empathetic understanding of the motivations, priorities and rationality of those studied. Without seeing things 'through the eyes' of the insider, the researcher will never be able to understand fully their perspective. This is vital, particularly in applied work that seeks to intervene in health behaviour. An 'insider' perspective provides access to the logic and rationality of what might seem at first merely misguided or irrational beliefs. Thus, in reading Victor Turner's work on Ndembu rituals, we come to understand how the Ndembu attribute misfortunes such as illness to various kinds of ritual transgressions, spirits and witches. Female reproductive troubles, for instance, are believed to result from the actions of the spirits of dead relatives. Rather than being merely random superstitious beliefs, ideas about the causes of particular symptoms and the appropriate remedies tie into an overarching cosmology that 'makes sense' of the misfortunes that afflict individuals from time to time. Although Turner notes that the ritual therapies used by the Ndembu may not be effective in public health terms (Turner 1967: 356), his ethnographic account provides a rich account of how they work at the social level, through reintegrating the sick person into society, for instance, or dealing with conflicts within the community.

However, without the 'stranger from Mars' perspective, such accounts will be limited. In everyday life, most of us have experience of having to 'learn the culture' of a new setting and become an insider. Starting a new college, or moving to a new country, entails learning all kinds of everyday rules about social behaviour and we are usually anxious to do this as quickly as possible to reduce the embarrassment of being an obvious novice or newcomer. In a research setting this process of social learning has to be made explicit, and the researcher reflects on how the rules were learned and what their significance is. Michael Agar (1980) uses the phrase 'professional stranger' to describe this role. If the fieldwork is protracted, the researcher has to guard against 'going native' and being merely a participant in the field, rather than an active participant observer. The 'stranger' element of the role has to be consciously maintained, in order to be able to ask the naïve question and analyse social life from a theoretical perspective.

Doing ethnography close to home

Early anthropologists studied alien cultures, largely small-scale societies in colonized African and Asian countries, in which the key challenge was to make the unfamiliar familiar. More recently anthropologists have turned their attention closer to home, with African and Asian researchers criticizing the misinterpretations of earlier generations (Fahim 1982) and those from the industrialized world focusing on the familiar as well as the 'other' with an ethnographic approach. Some examples of ethnographic methods used in industrialized settings include:

- *Studies of 'lay' health beliefs*. Cecil Helman (1978), for instance, looked at folk models of chills, fevers and colds in a North London suburb, and Charlie Davison and colleagues (1991) used ethnographic methods to look at lay epidemiological understandings of heart disease in South Wales.
- *Studies of health service organization and delivery*. Norman Fineman (1991) used observational and interview data to look at how clinicians, social workers and alcohol counsellors in a clinic constructed 'non-compliance' in the clients. Catherine Pope (1991) used observations and other methods to understand how waiting lists remain a problem for hospitals in the UK despite policy initiatives aimed at reducing them. David Hughes (1989) carried out a ten-month ethnographic study of an Accident and Emergency department, using the data to look at discretion in the work of reception and other non-clinical staff.
- *Cultural studies of biomedicine itself*. Deborah Lupton (1994) and Deborah Gordon (1988) have both used anthropological approaches to look at 'medicine as culture', and several anthropologists have analysed specific biomedical disease and epidemiological categories using the same approaches used for 'folk' categories.

In these studies using participant observation methods in studying industrialized health care settings, health professionals are often in a position of researching their own profession. Nurses, for instance, have carried out many studies of nursing care based on ethnographic methods for data collection. This poses particular methodological problems for maintaining a productive balance between insider and outsider perspectives and in making the familiar 'strange'. The advantages are clearly that access is much easier, and the researcher is already familiar with the emic perspective. Also, professional practice has provided a rich seam of potential research questions, and a good understanding of the feasibility of researching them. However, such 'insider' researchers face a far greater challenge in gaining analytical distance from their data, and may have to work much harder to treat the data theoretically. Jocelyn Lawler, in her work on the body in nursing (Lawler 1991), reflects on how this balance can be successfully achieved. As a nurse, Lawler was interested in the 'invisibility' of nursing work, and began thinking of how this could be related to the 'private' nature of much of the work they did caring for patients' bodies. She notes that although the physical body is taken for granted in everyday life, it becomes the focus of nursing work, and yet there is a relative absence of any 'talk' about it. She discusses the methodological challenges of researching 'taken for granted knowledge' and getting nurses to discuss explicitly what are not only taboo and sensitive issues, but ones that practitioners may have no adequate language to describe. Lawler argues that her 'insider' status was an advantage, even essential, to carrying out research on nursing:

> Because nursing is heavily influenced by experience, the researcher must share the same professional experience in order to decide what questions to ask nurses, if indeed the researcher wishes to get at the very essence of nursing practice. . . . One persistent feature of research involving nurses' work is the extent to which researchers have asked the 'wrong' questions. (Lawler 1991: 6)

For Lawler, then, an adequate insider understanding is an essential precondition for valid analysis, and she claims that professional experience is necessary to develop this. However, this is not a sufficient condition. She also drew on a combination of theoretical literatures to 'make sense' of the problem of the body, and articulate the 'taken for granted' knowledge of practitioners. This included a historical review of conceptualization of the body, literature on nursing and 'surveillance' of the body, and feminist approaches to the body and sexuality. This helps to maintain an analytical distance, but Lawler (by suggesting that only nurses can ask the 'right' questions) is situating herself firmly on the 'emic' end of the continuum, where faithfulness to the participants' own priorities and frameworks are key to validity.

Overt and covert roles

Overt roles are those in which the researcher is open about their role, whereas covert roles involve the researcher being 'under cover'. Most ethnographers are, to some extent, open about their role, but of course there are many potential ways to present your role in the field, and many interpretations people in the field will put on your account. Researchers working in areas where people are unfamiliar with the concept of research, or anthropology, are likely to be seen cast in more familiar roles by the host community – as spies or government officials, perhaps. One example comes from Richard Burghart's (1993) reflections on early fieldwork in his research on how people in Janakpur, in south-eastern Nepal, used the wells that still supplied water for some residents, and how they kept the water pure. He discusses how one community, the Cobblers, who were using a hand-pump in a neighbouring community as their well water was no longer 'sweet', originally assumed he had a rather more powerful role than merely that of a visiting researcher. He explained to a gathering crowd that he was there to learn from them how the well had lost its 'sweetness' and what they proposed to do to cure it, but heard members of the crowd repeating a rather different account to each other:

> The Cobblers ... turned to explain to newcomers ... that the government had told the sahib to tour the country and see the condition of the common people, and that my government was going to help the Cobblers clean the well. ... I quickly corrected them, saying I had not come from Kathmandu [i.e. from the Nepalese government] ... rather I had come from London. ... The inner circle now explained to the outer that I had been sent by the London government to tour Nepal to report on the condition of common folk. Now the British government were going to help them clean their well. ... I attempted to explain my ethical neutrality, political impartiality, indeed the objectivity of scientific research. Again, confusion spread throughout the crowd. (Burghart 1993: 82–3)

Burghart realized that his attempt to stress his impartiality has misfired completely, as local residents then assumed he was, in the eyes of the villagers, the worst of all visitors – a political broker, whose only function could be to play the two governments off against each other. In the event, he settled for an identity of a minor 'Lord', who would help the residents to purify their well.

In an unfamiliar setting, it may be impossible to predict how the community will interpret the role of the researcher. Even when the research setting is in a familiar culture, the researcher has to consider assumptions that will be made about their position, and who they are while doing fieldwork. Professionals working in familiar settings may be assumed to be 'experts', and those funded by government departments may be assumed to be working to a political agenda.

If trying to explain the role of the researcher brings problems, covert research, in which the researcher does not tell the community what they are doing, brings even more. Lawler's 'insider' status provided her 'cover' for much opportunistic observational work as she carried out normal duties, such as hospital-based teaching. However, she notes that these activities meant her role was more 'participant' than observer, and allowed little time for sustained observation. A longer-term period of observation was provided, also opportunistically, by the admission of a friend to hospital. Lawler thus had a legitimate role as a hospital visitor, allowing her to observe nursing work covertly. She notes:

> While I was aware of the ethical considerations inherent in using this situation for collecting data, I was also legitimately in the field as a visitor, and it was inevitable that I would find this time rich in ideas and data, and that it would contribute to my thinking on the ways in which nurses manage other people's bodies. I took advantage, opportunistically, of a naturally occurring event. (Lawler 1991: 13)

We discussed in Chapter 3 the ethical dilemmas involved in this kind of work, in which the role of the researcher is not disclosed to those in the field. Lawler's justification here is twofold: first, she wanted access to an 'undisturbed' natural environment in which the nurses' behaviour was not changed in response to a known observer (1991: 12). Second, as she notes above, it is very difficult to draw the line in long-term observational research between research and non-research activity. Health care is a diffuse activity, and we shall inevitably come across instances of our areas of interest in our everyday life. It would be impossible to discount all these stories and comments by friends and colleagues that might contribute to our eventual analysis, just because they weren't gained through a formal interview in which informed consent was sought. In addition, the meetings we have with potential gatekeepers, discussions with collaborators and observations made opportunistically while carrying out 'normal' activities such as visiting hospitals all provide 'data', which cannot be forgotten just because it was not a formal part of the data set. Even if never quoted in a report, these encounters, at a time when we are explicitly reflecting on a particular issue, are bound to influence the development of ideas. They should be treated with exactly the same critical awareness as other, more formal data, and as a valuable aid to the 'sociological imagination'.

These opportunistic observations are, though, arguably rather different from extended periods of 'covert' research, in which data collection is the primary goal, but no attempt is made to secure informed consent from participants or be explicit about the research role. As Chapter 3 discussed, this kind of research cannot be undertaken lightly, and must be justified by the impossibility of gaining data in other ways and the likely 'public interest' value of data gained. One covert observational strategy for data collection that has been widely used in health services research is the 'pseudo-patient study', deriving from market research 'mystery shopping'.

'Mystery shopping' and pseudo-patient studies

Mystery shopping is a technique taken from market research, involving the testing of services by researchers pretending to be 'real' consumers in order to find out how consumers are treated by service providers in everyday, rather than research, situations. As a form of covert observation, it has been used in health research, although not often by this name. Martin Bulmer (1982) uses the term 'pseudo-patient' studies to cover research that involves researchers pretending to be patients in order to find out how services are 'really' provided. As he notes, such strategies are used by investigative journalists and consumer organizations to 'test' services, as well as by researchers. There are a number of examples of such studies. Rosenhan's (1973) study of psychiatric hospitals, described in Case Study 3.2, is a classic, and mental health institutions have attracted many covert studies. Other health service topics researched by pseudo-patients include homeless people's access to primary health care in a

London borough (Hinton 1994), the differences between biomedical and Ayurvedic physicians in Sri Lanka (Waxler-Morrison 1988) and the routines of an acute hospital ward in Ghana (van der Geest and Sarkodie 1998).

Studies such as Rosenhan's are qualitative sociological studies of health care, in that they rely on ethnographic accounts from the pseudo-patients for their data. These covert methods are now not much used in sociological studies, largely because of the ethical problems involved. The need for informed consent from research participants in most settings means that many ethics committees would be unlikely to approve such a study. However, in health services research, there have been recent uses of pseudo-patients in evaluations of health care provision. Possibilities for securing consent include asking for consent retrospectively, and asking professional organizations to consent on behalf of their members. In these cases, the pseudo-patient is likely to only have a brief encounter with a provider, rather than an extended period in, say, a mental hospital. Here, the method is used more quantitatively, and perhaps in an experimental design. Hinton's (1994) study of access to primary care, for instance, compared how often actors playing three different people (a homeless rough sleeper, a Kurdish refugee and a middle-class woman) successfully registered as patients in 30 primary care surgeries. In Waxler-Morrison's (1988) study comparing Ayurvedic and biomedical physicians, trained research assistants presented standard symptoms and recorded standard information about their visit and the medicines prescribed. In these experimental designs, the qualitative data on experiences of health care may contribute to the study, but the major aim is to generate comparative quantitative data. Waxler-Morrison (1988), for instance, compared the number of times Ayurvedic and biomedical physicians carried out various investigations, volunteered particular information and prescribed Western or Ayurvedic medicines.

Madden et al. (1997) argue that these more quantitative pseudo-patient studies – or what they term *simulated client studies* – are a practical, feasible and economical method for researching health service provision in developing countries. For measuring actual practice, these methods provide better data than interviewing, as there are no problems with recall or social desirability bias, and better information than patient records, which may be inadequate. Reviewing studies that used simulated patients in developing countries, they note that they have been used to investigate a range of research questions, including evaluating training interventions, comparing pharmacy sales, and family-planning services. Although the main outcomes of these studies are quantitative, qualitative analysis might be used to examine issues such as communication in health care settings.

Following the ethical guidelines of the Council for International Organizations of Medical Sciences (CIOMS 1991), Madden et al. argue that provider consent may not be necessary if this would frustrate the purpose of the study. Despite noting that all researchers should be bound by the ethical norms of their own communities as well as those they study, they rather disconcertingly argue that weaker research governance is an advantage in developing countries, making pseudo-patient studies easier to conduct in these settings without consent: 'Government oversight tends to be weak, and there may be a general lack of labor/professional organizations, rights consciousness, and understanding of research. In many developing countries, social norms emphasize community rights over an individual's rights' (Madden et al. 1997: 1479).

Like all covert methods, pseudo-patient studies do raise particularly difficult ethical issues, particularly if (as Madden et al. are suggesting) the norms around consent may be different in the researcher's own institution and the fieldwork site. As we discussed in Chapter 3, a study to which participants cannot give informed consent is problematic. Justifications tend to focus on the high validity of data; the 'public interest' value of uncovering the real workings of health services, particularly in areas where patients may not be well served, such as mental health; and necessity – that such information can't be gathered in any other way. As the identity of the researcher is unknown to those in the field, the data gathered are uncontaminated by any researcher effects. Thus, if 'real' patient accounts are difficult to come by, or unlikely to be treated as 'valid', then the use of pseudo-patient studies may be the only way to generate convincing data on important topics such as discrimination in health service delivery. Aside from the substantial ethical problems, Martin Bulmer (1982) also argued that there are methodological problems. First, they encroach on the mutual trust and confidentiality of the 'real' doctor–patient relationship and involve deception. This can lead to a breakdown in trust between researchers and professionals. Second, there is the possibility of harm to the researcher if given unnecessary medical treatment, or stressed by their experiences. Third, even the claim to greater validity might be flawed, as real patients (if not professionals!) may be adept at identifying 'pseudo-patients' and presumably alter their behaviour in response.

Planning a participant observation study

So far, we have discussed in some detail the implications of various fieldwork roles (participant, participant-observer; stranger, insider; overt, covert) adopted by the researcher. Reflection on the methodological implications of the role is vital in thinking through the particular challenges of fieldwork (will it be learning the language? maintaining an analytical distance?), but there may be little leeway for choosing to adopt another role. Other decisions about participant observation studies present choices, and need considerable thought before embarking on the project. Some of the practical methodological implications of participant observation studies that should be considered are identifying a site, gaining access, refining observational skills, and approaches to recording data. These are all affected by both the specific setting of the proposed research and the nature of the researcher's role within it. To some extent, decisions about, for instance, how best to take notes will be determined by those necessities of the field that can only be known once there, but they are issues that should be thought through at the outset to minimize potential problems.

Identifying a site

Traditionally, ethnographic work is based on an in-depth study of one site, and issues of generalizability are conceptual rather than empirical. In Chapter 4, we suggested that sampling in qualitative interview work is often orientated towards generating 'information-rich' (Patton 1990) cases. This is true when selecting a single or small number of sites, which may be chosen because they typify some larger population of sites (such as clinics, or villages) or perhaps because they are exceptional in some way. Often, site selection is in practice a pragmatic decision, based on existing networks of colleagues and contacts. Paul Atkinson (1995) discusses how he ended up researching haematology, despite intending to investigate the interface between clinical and laboratory issues in pathology. Following a meeting at a conference in which he outlined his research interests to a colleague, the colleague then negotiated for him access to a teaching hospital in the United States with an honorary hospital appointment – an opportunity too good to pass up. The pathologists he approached were less receptive than the haematologists, and in the end the study focused only on haematology. In health services research, though, participant observation methods may be used across multiple sites, and care should be taken to select ones that represent a range of typical settings. Here, the researcher may be responsible for 'cold calling' potential sites to collaborate, rather than relying on informal sponsors within organizations.

Gaining access: the role of gatekeepers

Gatekeepers are those people who control access to the site and the people within it. They include formal gatekeepers whose permission is needed before fieldwork can commence (such as hospital managers, government departments or consultants) and informal gatekeepers, without whose support fieldwork will be impossible in practice. The formal gatekeepers depend on the setting, and the appropriate people must be identified early on. For work in institutional settings (such as hospitals or health agencies) the formal gatekeepers will be fairly easily identifiable. Introducing yourself 'cold', for instance by writing to Chief Executives or senior managers in the prospective sites, can be a very difficult strategy, and it is often advisable to use personal and professional networks to smooth the way. If you can be introduced as a friend or colleague, prospective gatekeepers have some way of 'placing' you socially, and are likely to be more trusting. However, 'cold' calling can work. Van der Geest and Sarkodie, in their small-scale participant observation study of a Ghanaian hospital, wrote to the secretary of the nearest hospital, and were surprised by a very positive response: the hospital considered it an honour to be chosen. This was contrary to the previous experience of van der Geest in Western countries, where there may be more reluctance to letting unknown social scientists in to observe.

In community settings, it can be more difficult to identify the appropriate formal gatekeepers, and those with extensive knowledge of the setting should be consulted. Organizations for indigenous peoples now often have formal policies for collaborating with research, which outline the proper channels of communication and approval. As one example, the Hopi people in Arizona, North America, have a protocol for 'research, publications and recording' which requires proposals for studies to be sent to the Office of Historic and Cultural Preservation for review and approval, and for prospective researchers to outline how the Hopi tribe will benefit from the study, and how consent from participants will be addressed (HCPO 2001). In other settings the process may be less formal, but there are usually some gatekeepers who must give their permission before any fieldwork can commence.

Informal gatekeepers are just as important, in that the researcher is reliant on their goodwill to carry out the study, but can be harder to identify before setting out on fieldwork. Paul Atkinson (1995: 16) discusses an early problem in his study of haematologists. Although access had been negotiated with the hospital Chief of Staff and senior staff in the department, he had not had time to meet with more junior staff before commencing. One was initially hostile, and complained about his presence. Although Atkinson managed to resolve the problem by writing to all staff reiterating that he had no interest in evaluating their work or of intruding, these kinds of problems can completely undermine fieldwork.

Refining observational skills

Learning to 'observe' analytically is a skill that takes time to develop; it is not just a matter of looking and recording, but of knowing what to look for and how to reflect on what is seen. For William Foote Whyte, a foundational assumption is that 'human behaviour is not random . . . but socially structured, and we need to discover the framework for such structuring' (Whyte 1984: 83–4). This is not, he suggests, a matter of looking at formal structures (such as organizational hierarchies or workplace divisions of labour) but looking at the regularities in social behaviour. Initial observations should be empirical: the idea is to describe what is going on, who is included, where it goes on and how, rather than one's 'impressions' or 'feelings' about the setting. This can be difficult to get started on, as any social field is a complex of many different activities and interactions. If it is an unfamiliar social setting, we may be tempted to impose our own assumptions of 'what is going on' from superficial similarities with those of our experiences. If the setting is a familiar one, it may be difficult to lose our professional frameworks for seeing what is happening. In Box 6.1 are John Lofland's (1971) suggestions for one way of dividing up 'the field' for observation.

Under each of the headings in Box 6.1, Lofland suggests that the researcher focuses on both static and 'phased' processes (that is, those that endure as features of a field, and those that change over time), either regularly or over

---

Box 6.1   Lofland's headings for organizing observations

Acts: brief occurrences of action
Activities: of longer duration
Meanings: verbal accounts that participants use to define what is going on
Participation: holistic involvement of participants in particular sets of acts
  and activities
Relationships: who is involved, and with whom
Settings: descriptions of whole sites

Source: Lofland (1971: 15).

---

the process of some change. One aim is to develop typologies for these different aspects of phenomena, by looking at how acts, activities and meanings are classified by those being studied. To take an example, if the fieldworker was beginning a period of observation of a community health clinic, they may begin by looking at the waiting room. Here, they might observe how patients wait (an *act*) for treatment, what they do while waiting in the waiting room (*activities*), who 'organizes' the queue for the doctor (*participation*), what communication there is between staff and patients in the waiting room (*relationships*), and what staff say their aim is in organizing the waiting area in a certain way (*meanings*). Putting together their observations of this and other phenomena, they can begin to build up a picture of the whole setting.

Note that 'observation' also includes, usually, talking to participants. 'Meanings' can only be elicited from asking people what acts or interactions mean to them. As well as people, the researcher observes space and material objects. How is the space of the clinic divided up, and how are these different spaces used? Who goes where, and when? Do people behave differently in different places, for instance taking off their uniforms when 'backstage' in the staff kitchen, or using formal titles to address each other when in public spaces?

Recording observations

Related to the issue of developing skills in observing is that of learning to record observations, and managing what can quickly become a large mass of data. The particular setting will determine to a large extent how observations are recorded, in terms of whether it is possible to make notes whilst observing (if on the less participant end of Gold's scale, or in an environment where writing notes will not seem 'odd') or whether the 'participant' role means that notes have to be written up at the end of each period of observation. But time to do this needs to be built into time in the field. One rule of thumb is to write up as soon as possible: at the end of the day, it is possible to remember most of the salient exchanges and decipher hurriedly scrawled notes; by the following day, these may be illegible and their salience forgotten. Tape recorders can be used to record opportunistic interviews, or a dictaphone to record observations for later transcription. It is good practice to keep separate empirical observational notes and your own initial interpretations, analytic comments and views, by using different notebooks, or colours. A fieldwork diary is essential for recording all aspects of the project, from early attempts to gain entry to the field and negotiations with gatekeepers to later reflections on the process.

Rapid ethnographic methods

As the examples so far in this chapter suggest, a key limitation of ethnographic work is that it is very time-consuming, taking many months for a researcher to gain access to a field, and to live or work there until their presence goes largely unnoticed. Agar reports that it usually takes about three months until he feels 'a functioning, accepted member of the community' (1980: 108). Meyer (1993) reports that her action research study of lay participation in care took six months to arrange access, one year of fieldwork and then six months of follow-up work, as she felt she could not withdraw from the field without consolidating the project. Turner's (1967) study of rituals in Ndembu society was based on two and a half years' fieldwork. This kind of extended study is typical of PhD studies in anthropology, but few researchers have the time to devote to such long-term participant observation later in a career. Additionally, few funding agencies are willing to take the risk of supporting a study that may have few clear aims at the beginning, and no guarantee of answering the research question first identified.

One attempt to preserve the advantages of observational work with feasibility in terms of resources is the development of so-called 'rapid' ethnographic methods, such as Rapid Rural Appraisal, Rapid Assessment Procedures and Participatory Rural Appraisal (Rifkin 1996). These are controversial, with some claiming that brief incursions into a field are likely to collect superficial or even misleading information. Agar (1980), for instance, discusses his experience of carrying out a survey during the early stages of fieldwork in Pakistan. Only later in his research did he realize how unreliable the early data were. People had assumed he was either a spy or a government agent, and had under-reported both young males in the household and their land holdings. In their study of beliefs about leprosy among the Limba of Sierra Leone, Opala and Boillot (1996) also doubt that less intensive methods would have identified what the causes of leprosy were from the perspective of the Limba. Reporting how the Limba avoid discussing witchcraft openly, they note how in interviews respondents feign ignorance completely, or make oblique references that would only be recognized by other Limba. In interviews, early responses to questions about the causes of leprosy included 'God's will', insect vectors and infected water. Only careful questioning from an interviewer with a grasp of Limba world-views unearthed deeply held, but rarely voiced, beliefs that leprosy was caused by witchcraft or as retribution for the evil done by a family member. More importantly, from a public health perspective, the researchers found that although most Limba saw modern medicines as effective against leprosy, few saw the early signs (red patches on the skin) as signs of leprosy, but rather saw it as a different disease, with different causes, and thus delayed seeking treatment until late in the disease progression. From a detailed anthropological understanding of Limba world-views, Opala and Boillot were able to work with health educators to shape public health messages about leprosy in ways that would mesh with the community's health beliefs. They suggest that programmes should employ a local anthropologist, even if they are not experts in medical anthropology, wherever possible to maximize the opportunities for in-depth understanding of how ideas about health and illness are embedded in local world-views.

These examples suggest that rapid appraisal may do more harm than good, through identifying 'public' accounts of health beliefs that are given to strangers, rather than more deeply held beliefs that are more likely to impact on health behaviour. However, rapid methods have proved useful in informing many public health interventions, and when carried out with care can generate useful data to aid specific projects. Susan Rifkin (1996) points to the advantages: relatively quick and cheap data collection and data that are addressed to designing practical interventions rather than academic findings. She reviews the origins of Rapid Rural Appraisal in the field of agriculture and rural development as a method for improving on existing surveys and other fact-finding techniques that were inadequate for decision-making. More recent approaches have incorporated a participatory element, with communities involved in the information collection and analysis. The resulting techniques of Rapid Participatory Appraisal have been widely used for health needs assessment both in developing and industrialized countries, and the World Health Organization publishes a guidebook on how to carry them out (Annett and Rifkin 1995).

Only data directly related to the project are collected, and the data collection methods come from a 'toolbox' of qualitative techniques, including interviews and various kinds of 'visualizations'. Visual representations are important not only when working in non-literate communities, but also because they are a good basis for discussion, and can generate information that does not come from an interview. Some of the data collection techniques in the 'toolbox' are illustrated in Box 6.2.

Care must be taken with choosing key informants to interview, to ensure that they can represent the interests of the whole community, and not just sectional interests. In the rapid appraisal approach, triangulation between these different sources of data aids validation.

The kind of data that this kind of 'rapid' ethnographic study produces, then, can, if done carefully, improve the effectiveness of public health interventions. Carl Kendall and colleagues discuss an attempt to widen access to oral rehydration therapy in Honduras through informing local people about the appropriate use of packets of oral rehydration salts (Kendall et al. 1984). Ethnographic studies suggested that one form of diarrhoea, called *empacho*,

---

Box 6.2   Examples of techniques from the Rapid Appraisal Toolbox

- Interviews with key informants such as:
  government officials, teachers, traditional healers, community leaders, shop owners.
- Visualizations such as:
  Seasonal calendars. Participants use illustrations to describe seasonal changes. These can be used to map disease prevalence, or household income, over different parts of the year.
  Mapping. Local materials (sand, pebbles) can be used by participants to create spatial maps of the locality, with access to resources marked, or changes over time illustrated.
- Observations
  of the physical environment, transport access, sanitation facilities, housing.
- Reports and other documents.

Sources: Rifkin (1996), Annett and Rifkin (1995).

---

was seen as caused by eating the wrong kinds of foods, and treatable by massage and purgatives. However, this information was not taken up in the campaign to inform people about oral rehydration salts. The campaign did not mention *empacho*, because programme staff did not see it as a 'real' disease entity in the way biomedical classifications are, and because they were uncomfortable with the idea of oral rehydration salts being promoted as a 'purgative'. Ignoring this folk classification meant that in the evaluation of the project, although local residents reported higher knowledge of oral rehydration therapy, they were unlikely to have used it in cases diagnosed as *empacho*. However, it is not enough for ethnographic information to exist, it must also be seen as reliable and relevant information by programme planners. Rapid appraisal is thus best conducted within a multi-disciplinary programme setting in which the findings can contribute to interventions. Case Study 6.1 is an example, from a programme designed to reduce the morbidity from diarrhoeal disease.

Rapid appraisal methods, then, offer a way of utilizing the insights of medical anthropology without the cost of in-depth ethnographic fieldwork. To be effective, however, these methods need using with care, and ideally with the help of local people who are fully conversant with the beliefs of the community. Such techniques are only 'rapid' in contrast with traditional ethnography; they are not a 'quick and dirty' way of doing social research for health.

Non-participant observational methods

At the 'complete observer' end of Gold's continuum are those methods in which the researcher does not have to be present in the field, or at least does not participate in the field. They are, perhaps, more associated with quantita-

---

Case Study 6.1   Applied anthropology in a diarrhoeal disease control project

(Source: Scrimshaw, S. and Hurtado, E. (1988) 'Anthropological involvement in the Central American diarrheal disease control project', *Social Science and Medicine*, 27: 97–105)

Susan Scrimshaw and Elena Hurtado note the importance of a detailed understanding of local health beliefs, culture and language for effective health interventions. In introducing oral rehydration therapy (ORT), for instance, it is vital to know local terms for different kinds of diarrhoea in order to target health promotion effectively, and to understand local health beliefs about both the causes and potential cures. Anthropologists have a large role to play in planning health interventions, through presenting data on folk health beliefs to public health specialists. As a contribution to a programme on reducing the morbidity from diarrhoeal disease in Central America, they collated ethnographic information on 'ethnoclassifications' of diarrhoea in four communities in Guatemala and Costa Rica. These proved to be complex. One taxonomy, from a highland community in Guatemala, included eight main kinds of diarrhoea, based on the primary cause: the mother, food, tooth eruption, fallen fontanelle or stomach, evil eye, stomach worms, cold or dysentery. These primary classifications were further subdivided. Different therapies were appropriate for different causes. Thus, if diarrhoea is caused by the mother being overheated (from pregnancy or being out on a hot day) and her milk being spoilt, the remedy would be to abstain from breastfeeding or weaning the baby. The only type of diarrhoea that was seen as appropriate to take to the clinic was that of dysentery, which was the most serious form and distinguished by blood in the stools. Others were seen as amenable to home cures (such as herbal teas, baths and massages) and various traditional healers. The ethnoclassifications of other communities differed in detail, but all included multiple types of diarrhoea with their own symptoms and preferred remedies. Explanations and therapies often combined biomedical and folk beliefs.

The implications for project planners are: that ORT has to be available widely in the community, through pharmacies and other stores, rather than only from the health clinic; that any information has to stress both the different kinds of diarrhoea in the local folk classifications and terminology; and that the need for rehydration in less serious categories of diarrhoea must be stressed. There is also scope for testing the effectiveness of home remedies identified, so that effective ones can be recommended.

To inform public health interventions, Scrimshaw and Hurtado recommend training project workers to carry out rapid ethnographic assessments in local communities to aid understanding of local health beliefs. They stress the need to present anthropological findings in ways that workers from other disciplines can understand. So rather than producing monographs using anthropological language, they summarize ethnoclassifications briefly as taxonomies, with diagrams if possible.

tive techniques in health research, in which observations are used to count and analyse behavioural phenomena. One example is a study of adverse events in hospitals (Andrews et al. 1997) which used trained ethnographers to observe ward rounds and meetings to identify all discussions of adverse events. The researchers did not ask questions, but just observed and collected standardized data on each event. However, non-participant observation offers great potential for qualitative analysis as well. Naturally occurring data are perhaps underused in health research, but can often be gathered fairly quickly, and with less disruption for the working life of a clinic or hospital. Audio, or even video, tape recordings of professional–client consultations are a useful source for research questions on communication in health care settings. Again, they have often been used in a more quantitative way, for instance by looking for the number of questions asked by each participant, or the length of time spent on aspects of the consultation, but there is also the potential for ethnomethodological analysis.

Developed by the sociologist Harold Garfinkel (1967), 'ethnomethodology' means 'folk methods' and refers to the rules and processes by which people give meaning to behaviour and interpret social interaction. Garfinkel's focus was on the micro-level of social life: how interaction gets accomplished, and what potentially disrupts it. Although this branch of sociology has been criticized for being overly concerned with the minutiae of interpersonal communication, rather than broader questions of social structure, it clearly has a valuable contribution to our understanding of health care, where interpersonal communication is a key element. Of particular interest in areas of health care such as primary care and counselling, one aspect of communication is how well professionals allow patients or clients to 'tell their story', both to allow access to diagnostic information and as a therapeutic device in itself (see Greenhalgh and Hurwitz 1998, for example, on the renewed interest in narratives in medicine). The research described in Case Study 6.2 takes an ethnomethodological approach to look at how story-telling does or does not get accomplished in clinical settings.

Detailed analysis of naturally occurring talk from settings such as hospital clinics provides a useful source of research on how health care communication happens in practice, as opposed to participants' accounts of it. Like other observational methods, the key strength is that it utilizes data about 'real' behaviour. Following Harvey Sacks (1989), David Silverman (1993: 51–5) argues that an ethnomethodological approach has advantages over other ethnographic approaches, as well as over interview data, potentially addressing methodological shortcomings such as the tendency to generalize from small extracts from a data set. The methodological advantages arise from a focus on empirical, observable detail (using, for instance, reproducible data from transcripts of naturally occurring talk, which can be studied by a number of analysts) and the 'topicalization' of common sense. The 'topicalization' of common sense means that the kinds of resources individuals in any setting draw on to make sense of their world (and that we, as researchers, use to

Case Study 6.2   Non-participant observation: using video-tapes to examine story-telling in consultations

(Source: Clark, J. and Mischler, E. (1992) 'Attending to patients' stories: reframing the clinical task', *Sociology of Health and Illness*, 14: 344–72)

Patients' stories are an important topic in research in physician–patient communication. Jack Clark and Elliott Mischler are interested in how story-telling does or doesn't happen in a clinical encounter: what interactional skills are needed by the physician, and how does a story get 'accomplished' in a particular encounter? The study uses data from video-tapes that are routinely taken for evaluation and training purposes in an out-patient clinic of a large teaching hospital in the United States. The clinic encourages patient-centred consultations. Two tapes were chosen for analysis: one that clinic staff thought exemplified a patient-centred consultation, and one that didn't. The video-tapes were transcribed in detail, with intonation, pauses and interruptions all transcribed. The two transcripts were then compared to identify the differences between them in terms of interaction. Although both patients had chronic illnesses and were from similar social backgrounds, and both clinicians had similar training, analysis revealed differences in how the initial problem is presented, how symptoms are determined and how therapeutic decisions are discussed.

In the first transcript, a man with epilepsy succeeds in 'telling his story': presenting a seizure he experienced in the context of his work as a car mechanic. His story 'embeds an illness event in the context of his lifeworld, combining personal knowledge, identity claims and relevant features of the everyday working life in which his illness is experienced' (p. 350). Whilst gathering the clinical details needed for the consultation, the physician collaborates in the story-telling by reiterating key points, pausing for continuation and acknowledging the relevant facts of the story. In contrast, the patient in the second video, a woman with diabetes, does not manage to 'tell her story', but instead presents a list of disconnected symptoms as the clinician shifts focus throughout her account to prompt for 'relevant' details, and ignores the context of her story. Her attempts to maintain the narrative are interrupted, and the physician misses the point she makes about her concerns. These differences in style continue through to the end stages of the consultation. In the first case, the physician collaborates with the man with epilepsy to request a blood sample (saying 'If it's okay with you I would like to have a blood test taken today. Is that all right?'). In the second, the physician announces his intention to do tests: 'We ought to check your sugar in the lab since you're here.' For Clark and Mischler, the importance of being able to 'tell a story' within a consultation relates to the need for patients to make sense of the physiological aspects of their illness in terms of its impact on the social fabric of their lives. Chronic illness, in particular, requires managing complicated treatment regimes whilst maintaining personal control. A consultation in which what the authors call 'the voice of the lifeworld' is heard is likely to lead not only to better patient satisfaction, but also to better control of illness for patients.

> From analysing transcripts of consultations, Clark and Mischler are able to identify different ways in which patients and physicians actually accomplish clinical work. A detailed look at how the clinical tasks of diagnosis, ordering tests and deciding on treatment are managed in practice allows them to focus on the skills of physicians, and the ways in which consultations can be carried out in a more 'patient-centred' way.

make sense of what we see in that world) are subject to analysis to see exactly how these understandings are accomplished, through focusing on what can be observed, rather than making assumptions about how categories or concepts are utilized and what they mean.

Thus, if studying, say, 'how doctors break bad news in a consultation', the researcher does not trawl the transcripts looking for examples of 'bad news' from a predetermined definition of what this would look like, or ask participants what they think about how 'bad news' is broken. Rather, detailed transcriptions are analysed to look for how both parties achieve the communication of news in the setting. How do patients register particular utterances as 'bad' or 'good'? How do the participants in the consultation use talk to achieve shared understanding of the meaning of a particular utterance? Geraldine Leydon (Leydon and Green 2001) used this approach to analyse how information was shared between cancer patients and their doctors in hospital outpatient clinics. By looking in detail at transcripts of consultations, she demonstrated how doctors skilfully lead up to 'breaking bad news' by first establishing what patients already know about their diagnosis, and by pairing 'good news/ bad news' statements such as 'we completely removed·the tumour [good] but found cancer cells in the lymph nodes [bad]'. Using conversation analysis, Leydon was able to focus in detail on what actually went on in the consultation, rather than relying on either patients' or doctors' accounts of information exchange.

Detailed analysis of naturally occurring data has been used productively in a number of health settings, largely in industrialized countries. Examples include:

- Douglas Maynard's (1991) study of consultations in paediatric clinics, which identified how doctors break bad news through careful monitoring of the parents' perspectives and knowledge first.
- Anssi Peräkylä and David Silverman (1991) looked at the organization of talk within HIV counselling interviews, examining the ways in which counsellors covered delicate topics, and used particular communication formats to achieve tasks such as delivering information about safer sex, advising the client and gaining consent for a test.
- Derrol Palmer (2000) analysed recorded interviews between hospital patients and clinicians to identify how 'delusional' talk was recognized in practice by professionals.

Conclusion

Qualitative observational methods include, then, traditional ethnographic approaches associated with anthropology, more recent developments of 'rapid' ethnographic methods, and detailed non-participant observational work on naturally occurring talk or behaviour. In health research, there has often been an assumption that observational data are 'better' and more valid than those produced by other methods (such as interviews, or official statistics). Although observational designs do have undoubted methodological strengths, they are not appropriate for all research questions, and may not be feasible for many research questions. However, some observational work is essential in most qualitative studies, even if only as 'background' to a particular research topic, or a way of assessing the feasibility of other designs in the study context. Brief periods of observational work (for instance, shadowing members of staff for a shift, or sitting in a clinic reception area) can be very productive for sensitizing researchers to issues to ask about in interviews, or learning about the constraints faced by research participants. The methods used by ethnographers have, for this reason, been adopted in a range of qualitative health studies, and most research designs benefit from some observational work.

Research designs that draw extensively on observation data are required for some research questions. If the concern is with the detailed analysis of particular settings in which transcriptions of talk are possible, then conversation analysis has been suggested as a reliable and valid method for studying how people actually interact in health care settings, rather than what they say they do. If the aim of the research is to really understand 'what is going on' in a particular setting in a holistic way, a long-term participant observation study, in which the researcher integrates both emic and etic perspectives, is the design of choice.

KEY POINTS
- The major strength of observational methods is that they provide data on what people do, as well as what they say they do.
- In ethnography, long-term participation in the field enables the researcher to capitalize on both distance and familiarity to analyse social behaviour.
- Doing ethnography in familiar sites has benefits in terms of access and familiarity, but poses challenges for the researcher in achieving analytic distance.
- Rapid ethnographic techniques have been widely used in public health research, with some success, although there has been debate about the validity of data generated.
- Non-participant observational methods provide access to social interaction with minimal intervention in the field and are one way of producing empirical and reliable data for analysis.

EXERCISES

1   Jocelyn Lawler argues that her 'insider' status was an advantage when researching nursing work. Consider a setting with which you are familiar (such as a workplace, neighbourhood, college). List the practical and methodological advantages and disadvantages of you carrying out an ethnography of this setting.

2   Carry out an observation of a public setting (such as a fast food restaurant or train station). Make notes on how different people in that setting behave, using the headings in Box 6.1 as a guide. You could consider: who uses the facility, how do they interact and with whom, how do they use space? Compare your observations with those of colleagues or classmates.

FURTHER READING

Agar, M.H. (1980) *The professional stranger: an informal introduction to ethnography*. San Diego: Academic Press. This is a readable account of the practical and methodological issues raised by doing traditional fieldwork.

Hammersley, M. (1992) *What's wrong with ethnography?* London: Routledge. A theoretical discussion of the methodological assumptions of 'ethnography', in which Hammersley argues that it is not a separate methodology. Covers issues such as generalizability, realism and theory in ethnographic work.

7

Using Documentary Sources

CHAPTER SUMMARY

It is not always necessary to collect new primary data for research, and using existing documents can be an efficient use of resources for many qualitative questions. Potential documentary sources include public records, private documents, research publications, archived research data and mass media sources. Like data produced by the researcher, documentary data can be analysed from a number of qualitative perspectives.

Introduction

We use the term 'documents' here to refer widely to the whole range of written sources that might be available relating to a topic, and by extension other artefacts that can be treated as documents. This is, of course, a rather disparate set of potential data sources. Those that have been used in qualitative health research studies include (among many others) newspapers, government reports, personal and work diaries, letters, research articles, primary data from other projects, job descriptions, organizational charts, manuals, medical records, films, photographs and medical instruments. Given both the range of documents that researchers could access, and the range of perspectives that researchers bring to them, it would be impossible to deal comprehensively with the practical and methodological problems raised by 'documentary research' as if it were a particular research strategy. Here, we address the possibilities of using existing documents instead of generating new primary data, and highlight how some of the most accessible sources of documents can be used for health research questions.

Why use existing sources?

All research of course relies on some analysis of documentary sources. At a minimum we have to review the existing research outputs in the relevant area, and perhaps draw on policy reports to make a case for the timeliness or policy relevance of our own research. Most qualitative projects also draw on a variety of documents in the field for background context on the setting, population or health problem addressed in the research. Case studies and ethnographic research will often draw widely on a variety of documentary sources in addition to data from interviews and observations, including perhaps reports from the organizations studied, diaries of research participants, or material artefacts used and produced in the setting. For some research projects this will be 'background' information, used only to orientate the researcher in refining the research question and design. In other studies, these documents and artefacts will be part of the corpus of data that will be analysed to answer the research question. Many research questions can be addressed by exclusively using existing sources of data, rather than by producing new data. There are a number of advantages in relying on available documents as the primary data source for research.

A first incentive for using documentary sources is their abundance and availability. Modern societies produce vast amounts of data, from official statistics such as censuses and surveys, birth, marriage and death certificates, to private records such as diaries, photographs and personal archives. In most countries, government departments and agencies devote considerable resources to collecting data about the population, and have the advantage of far greater resources than the academic researcher can ever muster. In addition to this 'official' record of our lives, many of us also produce throughout our lifetimes informal 'private archives' – data sources that ordinarily remain in the household, including photograph albums, letters and, more recently, videos and e-mail correspondence. These diverse sources are sometimes divided into *records*, which are produced to provide evidence of some transaction or event (such as marriage, or a hospital visit), and *documents*, which refers to those produced for personal rather than official purposes. Another existing data source comes from previous research studies. Increasingly, qualitative data generated as primary data for one study are being archived for use by other researchers (Backhouse 2002). Given the sheer volume of potential sources of data already in existence, researchers perhaps have to consider whether their study really justifies adding to this by producing yet more primary data.

A second reason to use documents is of course that for some research problems, documents will be the only source of data. For historical research, there may be no living people to interview, and we are reliant on witness accounts recorded at the time, and other contemporaneous records. In a study of nursing in Uganda, Pat Holden (1991), for instance, wanted to understand contemporary tensions in a Kampala hospital, in which working conditions and salaries for nurses were very poor, but in which nurses still turned up for work, often in 'beautifully laundered uniforms', despite water shortages and few obvious incentives. To explore the current situation, she traces the development of nursing during the colonial period, which she argues has left a legacy of nursing ideology that may be inadequate for the crisis conditions now faced by nurses in Uganda. In her research, Holden draws largely on documentary data, including the papers of the Overseas Nursing Association and reminiscences collected by another researcher as part of a project on public health services in Africa, as well as contemporary ethnographic data. Documents provide the data for exploring the history of nursing in Africa and the concerns of the nursing profession in the early part of the twentieth century.

Third, there are some not insignificant practical advantages. One relates to the preferences of the researcher. Some researchers may be far more comfortable with documents than people: not everyone has the aptitude or desire to develop the interactive skills needed for qualitative fieldwork or interviewing. Finally, projects based solely on publicly available sources are also unlikely to require ethical approval to conduct.

This chapter discusses potential documentary sources for research under four broad headings: public records, personal documents, mass media outputs and research outputs. Each of these can be utilized for health research studies from a number of theoretical perspectives, from positivist studies using research reports as data for an extended literature review to social constructionist studies using discourse analysis to analyse documents as texts. The type of document (whether mortality reports from the World Health Organization, or newspaper articles, or diaries) does not imply a particular methodological approach: like any other data source, the use to which they are put depends on the research question and the orientation of the researcher. The approaches given as examples under the headings of public records, personal documents, mass media outputs and research outputs are not, then, the only approaches that can be used with these types of data, but are intended as illustrations of the potential for using documents for health research.

Public records

Public records, or official statistics, are produced by international organizations (such as the World Health Organization and the World Bank), national governments and other agencies, and authorities such as health authorities. These data provide a rich source for quantitative secondary analysis (see Hakim 1982 for a discussion), and of course are often the source of new research questions, both qualitative and quantitative. Most qualitative studies will make use of these public records in some way, even if only in the literature review as part of the 'evidence' for the usefulness of the study proposed, or to document the characteristics of the population of interest. However, there are also a number of ways in which public records can be used as the primary data for qualitative research, as the topic for analysis. Indeed, official reports based on official statistics offer a rich seam for qualitative analysis. Social constructionists have inevitably made most use of these sources, as they provide an important longitudinal record of 'official' classifications of the social world, including that of health and medicine. What is of interest here is not the numbers reported (how many people died of cancer in this or that year, how many births this or that region had), but how they are categorized: how disease categories change over time, or what kind of illness episodes are officially reported. A social constructionist analysis of published data sets can address questions about what organizations consider it important to record at particular points in time, how this changes over time and space, and how the classification systems have changed. Case Study 7.1 is an example of this approach.

This kind of analysis has been a fruitful one for medical sociology, with a number of studies drawing on official statistics and reports to uncover the social construction of classification systems; see, for instance, Green's (1999) work on how the prevention of accidental injury has been constructed in public health discourse, or Sarah Nettleton's (1992) work on how the mouth has come to be stabilized and understood through the practice of modern dentistry. More recently, there has been an interest in including artefacts as well as written documents in these analyses, and focusing on technologies of classification (computer programs, statistical tests) as well as the texts (such as the International Classification of Diseases, or public health reports) that result from classificatory activity. One example is from Geoffrey Bowker and Susan Star (1999), who aimed to explore 'the creation and maintenance of complex classifications as a kind of work practice, with its attendant financial, skill and moral elements' (Bowker and Star 1999: 5). Looking in detail at the 10th revision of the International Classification of Diseases (ICD), which is the internationally used tool for classifying diseases for epidemiological work, they show how it is a pragmatic system, which has embedded in it a host of social factors. For instance, in looking at the detailed breakdown of categories for accidents there are a wide range of choices for various falls (from a cliff, from a wheelchair, from bed, from a commode, and so on) but very few for differentiating the kinds of accidents likely to happen in less industrialized areas of the world. Similarly, deaths from snake or spider bites can only be differentiated as those from venomous or non-venomous species. As Bowker and Star note:

Case Study 7.1   The social construction of Sudden Infant
Death Syndrome

(Source: Armstrong, D. (1986) 'The invention of infant mortality', *Sociology
of Health and Illness*, 8: 211–32)

David Armstrong's (1986) exploration of the emergence of Sudden Infant
Death Syndrome in Britain in the twentieth century is an example of the
use of official statistics to answer a research question about the social construction of the categories we use routinely in epidemiology. Tracing the
ways in which deaths of infants were classified, reported and analysed in
official reports, such as those of the Registrar General, Armstrong noted
that infant mortality rates were only reported from 1877 onwards. The statistical technology needed to calculate a mortality rate existed before then,
but only once infants had been recognized as a socially significant category
was a rate for their deaths reported. This illustrates well the kinds of questions a social constructivist asks of the data: not 'How did the rate of infant
death change over the nineteenth century?' but rather 'When, and why, did
it become possible to report on deaths of infants in this way?'

In the early twentieth century, the 'problem' of infant deaths, Armstrong
argues, moves from being a biological one to a social one with a growing
interest in the use of infant mortality as an indicator of the health of communities. It continues, of course, to be used in this way, particularly in international comparisons. The period of infancy became demarcated, with the
gradual establishment of 'neonatal' to mean the first four weeks of life,
and later a concentration on the first week of the neonatal period. There
was nothing inevitable about this: at various points in the nineteenth century, periods of two months and three months were used. Like other categories, they appear 'obvious' ones that we may be accustomed to using,
but an analysis of their emergence unpacks their social construction.

For Armstrong, these historical shifts observable in public records are not
necessarily evidence of the development of medical understanding of infant
deaths or the inevitable outcome of epidemiological analysis of those
deaths. Instead, the records and documents also create an object (in this
case, the infant) and can be analysed to demonstrate how that object is constructed. He argued that 'analysis and object are mutually constitutive:
that the infant is as much a product of the analysis as the analysis is a reflection of the infant' (Armstrong 1986: 227). In terms of the debates we
reviewed in Chapter 1 about the epistemological underpinnings of qualitative research, Armstrong is explicitly placing himself in the social constructionist camp, and rejecting the realist position that 'infants' have a pre-
existing stable reality.

> The ICD is richest in its description of ways of dying in developed countries at this moment in history: it is not that other accidents and diseases cannot be described, but they cannot be described in as much detail. . . . So the ICD bears traces of its historical situation as a tool used by public health officials in developed countries. (Bowker and Star 1999: 76)

Public records, then, as well as providing essential information from a positivist perspective, are also a rich source of data for those interested in exploring the ways in which the categories used in health and medicine are constructed. At a minimum, these kinds of studies remind health researchers that the taken-for-granted categories used in epidemiological research are socially constituted, rather than inevitable or natural ways of dividing up the world. Beyond that, qualitative analysis of official statistics can explore how political and social factors (such as the development of ICD to meet the public health needs of developed countries) shape the kinds of data that are collected and reported.

Personal documents

Historians have perhaps made the most use of personal documents, as resources such as diaries and letters are often the only available source of data to shed light on lived experience in anything other than the most recent history. However, personal documents are also a useful source of data for any project that addresses, or aims to include, a biographical perspective. Norman Denzin (1989a) argues that the biographical method (using autobiographical and biographical sources) has been seen in the social sciences as a way of incorporating the subjective experiences of individuals, and how they give meaning to their lives. He cautions against any simplistic notion that diaries and other autobiographical sources are in any way reflections of a 'real' self, as of course all biographies (even the most personal diary) are produced as stylized narratives, written for particular audiences using conventional structures. They are, he argues, essentially literary constructions, and must be analysed as such, with due regard to the symbolic use of language, the social functions the writing performed, and the acceptance that biographies represent partial identities and lives, not the whole truth about such lives.

Some classic studies widely cited in qualitative health research have drawn extensively on documentary sources. Erving Goffman's essay on *Stigma* (Goffman 1963), for instance, used a range of sources such as autobiographies, published diaries, examples from published studies and fiction to develop a sociological understanding of 'stigma' and its impacts on everyday social interaction. Goffman was interested in how discrediting attributes (such as disability, physical marks, or particular ethnic identities) disrupt the taken-for-granted aspects of interaction, and lead to damaged self-identities for those stigmatized. Given the wealth of existing sources of data, Goffman had no need to interview people, or undertake any extended observations to meet his aims, which were to 'review some work on stigma . . . to see what it can yield for sociology' (1963: 9).

Mass media outputs

Media outputs such as newspaper reports, television programmes and film provide an accessible source of data for many health research questions. Contemporary sources are easily collated or observed, and in many countries there are good newspaper and film archives. Media outputs, like public records and personal documents, can be used to address questions about the social construction of health and illness.

One example is Elina Oinas's (1998) work on menstruation, which used data from the medical advisory columns of ten Finnish magazines. She identified all the letters published in these columns, with the doctors' answers, that related to menstruation to explore how the issue of menstruation is medicalized. For this kind of topic, these kinds of documentary sources are an interesting data set – Oinas suggests that medical columns are one of the few public arenas in which menstruation is discussed. From her analysis of the letters and answers, she identifies the key concerns of (largely) young women: normality and dealing with the etiquette of menstruating. Through the letters and answers, Oinas suggests that the women writers and medical professionals construct a 'proper' role for medicine as the arbiter of normality, and the need for medical expertise to determine the nature of the body and to be responsible for its functioning.

A second perspective in studies of mass media output is analyses of how health issues are represented in the media. Given the importance of the media as an influence on public perceptions of health and illness, exploring these public images of health issues can shed light on how they are framed and what messages (intended and unintended) they convey. Often, studies of media representations combine quantitative and qualitative methods of analysis. A study by Lesley Henderson and colleagues (Henderson et al. 2000) of how infant feeding was represented in the British media, for instance, used quantitative content analysis of newspaper and television coverage to identify how often references were made to breast and bottle feeding and whether any problems were associated with the method. They found that breast feeding was rarely shown, and when it was it was often as problematic. Newspaper coverage often commented on potential problems with breast feeding, but rarely on its health benefits. Combined with this was a qualitative analysis of the contexts in which images of infant feeding occurred. This suggested that breast feeding was commonly associated with humorous story lines in fictional television programmes, and with middle-class or celebrity women. In contrast, bottle feeding was presented as largely invisible and associated with 'normal' families. Here, using documentary sources (national newspapers, a sample of television programmes) enabled the researchers to explore media representations of an important health issue in the UK, which has one of the lowest rates of breast feeding in Europe. Analysing representations suggested some influences on this health behaviour, in that breast feeding is portrayed as problematic and likely to fail whereas bottle feeding is represented as the normal and obvious choice.

Research outputs

In many ways, existing research outputs, whether primary data collected by other researchers or secondary sources (such as research reports and peer-reviewed journal articles), are the ideal source of data for projects when resources are limited. Primary data (typically, interview transcripts or diaries collected in the course of previous research) can be analysed to address new research questions, or re-analysed from new perspectives. Analysis of secondary sources is an efficient strategy for topics on which there has already been considerable previous research, as much can be gleaned by synthesizing existing research evidence.

Using existing primary data

The efficiency gains of re-analysis of primary data such as interview transcripts from other studies may be particularly important for small student projects where there is limited time or resources for new data collection. However, there has been encouragement for all researchers to consider this as a good strategy for exploiting previous research activity to the full. Increasingly, qualitative researchers are archiving their data for future re-analysis. In the UK, the Economic and Social Research Council requires all grant holders to archive their data if possible and funds a service (called Qualidata) for encouraging the archiving, dissemination and re-use of data, based at the University of Essex (www.qualidata.essex.ac.uk). These archives require data to be anonymized, and any identifying details to be removed.

Networks of supervisors and colleagues are another good source of readily available data. Most researchers feel that they have never exploited their own data fully, and may be happy for someone else to explore different themes in their data, or use it to address a new research question. The ethical implications of re-analysis for a different purpose need to be considered, particularly if consent was only sought from participants for one particular study.

Some data sources are specifically designed to be repeatedly 'mined' for further projects. One example is the British Mass-Observation Archive. This was originally commissioned in the 1930s as a project to gather everyday accounts of social life in Britain from volunteer observers. A new panel of observers was recruited in the 1980s, who are asked to write about aspects of their lives in response to 'directives' suggesting particular topics. Their accounts are then anonymized, so that they can be archived for future research. Helen Busby (2000) argues that these autobiographical sources of data offer potentially rich and fruitful insights into health and illness topics, particularly when the researcher is interested in subjective accounts of the interrelationships of health and other aspects of everyday life. Using the replies to a series of directives on topics such as staying well, the pace of life and doing a job, Busby is able to follow case studies of individuals and explore how work, family and leisure have an impact on their health, and how moral discourses of 'keeping going' are used to describe poor health that does not necessitate time off work. These kinds of archives provide, then, invaluable resources for future researchers.

Secondary analysis of research reports

Even more readily available are secondary sources, particularly published articles. These can be a rich source of material for studies using *discourse analysis*. The term 'discourse analysis' is utilized in a number of ways across the qualitative research literature (Potter and Wetherell 1987), but here we are using it to refer to those analyses of texts (including spoken language or artefacts that can be analytically treated as texts) orientated towards broad-ranging ideological explorations of how particular texts achieve their effects. The aim is to reveal how language (and indeed any other sign system, such as the uniforms of staff or the architecture of a hospital) does its work, in conveying not just the superficial meaning, but also the less obvious social meanings.

One example is from Patricia Kaufert (1988), who was interested in how the menopause is constructed through medical research. She looked at research reports on the topic of menopause not to review the findings, but to explore how these texts did their work of creating the discrete medical category of 'menopause'. Her data set includes: a 1985 review of current research, aimed at informing gynaecologists and general practitioners about the state of medical knowledge, published by two leading researchers in the field, plus the 122 original research publications included in their review. For each publication Kaufert classified the kind of study, how 'menopause' was defined, and the characteristics and size of the study population. There were three main categories of paper: epidemiological studies, clinical research and clinical case studies. She then analysed how the reviewers used these different materials in constructing their analysis. This included examining which sources were and were not used at various points, how they contributed to the overall argument of the review, and how important information in the original papers (such as the inclusion of 'artificially menopausal women' in the study population) was often missing from the review. A key element missing was any sense of women's own voices – the review included nothing on how women talked about experiencing the menopause. The research papers reviewed also had limited data on non-Caucasian populations, although patterns were reported as though universal. Kaufert's study is a good example of how this kind of secondary analysis can reveal the ways in which medical knowledge is produced, and how the 'facts' produced through specific methodological processes then come to have a life of their own as 'knowledge'.

Qualitative secondary analysis of research reports does not have to be in this social constructionist tradition. In Case Study 7.2, the data used for secondary analysis are also research reports, but they have been used in a rather more positivist way, to shed light on a health problem, that of post-partum depression in the US (Stern and Kruckman 1983).

In Case Study 7.2, the authors do not have a primary aim of exploring the *production* of these anthropological studies, or analysing them as texts, although they do of course take into account how they were produced, in pointing to the limitations of taking data collected for one purpose to address a new question. Rather, they are reviewing the findings reported to extend our understanding of post-partum depression. In health care, the idea of a *systematic review* of the literature as a way of synthesizing the findings from quantitative (especially RCT) studies has become popular recently, as an element of the move towards evidence-based medicine and health care (Petticrew 2001). There have been attempts to extend this kind of exercise to qualitative empirical studies, where the aim is to identify all relevant studies in the area, appraise their quality (see Chapter 11) and synthesize the findings from the methodologically sound studies in the review. However, there have been few published reviews of qualitative research that attempt this kind of systematic approach, partly because this model of secondary analysis is built on a rather positivist notion of research in which the empirical findings can be stripped from their production, and synthesized. Nicky Britten and colleagues (Britten et al. 2002) argue that there are good grounds for developing formal methods of meta-analysis for qualitative studies, as an alternative to traditional narrative reviews of existing literature, and suggest a more qualitative approach for doing this. Using George Noblit and R. Dwight Hare's (1988) strategy of *meta-ethnography*, they conducted a meta-analysis of published papers on lay meaning of medicines.

Essentially, meta-ethnography entails a re-analysis of the concepts that are reported in published studies on similar topics. The first set of concepts included in the meta-ethnography are those reported from the participants in the primary studies: these are called 'first-order concepts'. In the meta-ethnography reported by Britten and colleagues, these were: adherence/compliance; self-regulation; aversion; alternative coping strategies; sanctions; and selective disclosure. Second-order constructs are social scientific concepts that are reported as outcomes of the original analysis. In the papers on the meanings of medications, these second-order concepts included the impact of cultural meanings, and 'cost-benefit analysis'. The second-order interpretations are the building blocks for the meta-analysis, in which the researcher develops an argument about how they are linked, and attempts to synthesize the insights from all papers included in the review. Britten and colleagues did this with the aid of a grid, in which all the first- and second-order concepts are listed. Thus, they can develop a generalizable theory about medicine-taking, from integrating the findings and analysis of a number of published empirical papers on the topic. These final 'third-order' interpretations that form the synthesis are then potentially testable hypotheses. Part of their synthesis is as follows:

Case Study 7.2   Using ethnographic studies to shed light on post-partum depression

(Source: Stern, G. and Kruckman, L. (1983) 'Multi-disciplinary perspectives on post-partum depression: an anthropological critique', *Social Science and Medicine*, 17: 1027–41)

Gwen Stern and Laurence Kruckman are interested in a common syndrome in the United States, that of 'post-partum depression'. This mild and transient form of depression in mothers after the birth of a baby is very common, affecting 60–80 per cent of new mothers in Western countries, and is characterized by feelings of sadness, weeping, irritability and fatigue. Stern and Kruckman note that most research on this syndrome has focused on biological and psychosocial correlates and that there has been little attention to possible cultural factors such as the structure of the family or role expectations of the new mother. To explore the issue of cultural factors, they reviewed the ethnographic literature on childbirth. They found very little evidence of similar 'illnesses' affecting new mothers in non-Western settings. Studies from settings as diverse as Nepal, China, Nigeria and southeast Asia identified post-partum depression as a rare or absent disorder, although childbirth is recognized in most cultures as a significant life event.

They suggest that post-partum depression could be described as a culture-bound syndrome – an illness that takes a particular form in particular social settings. Turning to why it may be that so many women in the US suffer from the disorder, Stern and Kruckman draw on ethnographic descriptions of other culture-bound illnesses to suggest a relationship between perceptions of 'role helplessness' and mental illness. Specifically, they propose a relationship between the strategies available within a culture to support the new mother and her mental health. Compared with what is known from ethnographic studies of other settings, mothers in the US face a relative lack of social structuring of the post-partum period, little recognition of their role transition and little practical help. In many cultures, the post-partum period is typically a time of rest and vulnerability, in which the mother has to be protected and often secluded. This seclusion and rest is often facilitated by practical help from female kin in carrying out the mother's normal duties such as cooking, helping out with the household and looking after other children. Alongside the practical help, many cultural traditions entail emotional support for the mother. These might include washing her body or hair, the giving of gifts, ceremonial foods or massage. These traditional rituals mark the transition to a new role and act as a focus for social support for the new mother.

Using published ethnographic studies, then, Stern and Kruckman are able to demonstrate that post-partum depression is not a universal phenomenon. They are also able to suggest some cultural factors that may make women in Western countries particularly vulnerable by pointing to the range of traditional practices that protect the new mother in many non-Western societies. However, they also note some limitations in this approach. First, childbirth has only recently come to the attention of anthropology, so many ethnographies have little information on post-partum practices. Of those that do, few studies used formal diagnostic testing. Given the ambiguity over definitions of post-partum depression, this would also be difficult to do cross-culturally, given that the behavioural indicators, such as weeping, may well be culturally specific. They cannot, then, use these secondary sources to 'prove' their hypothesis about the cultural aetiology of post-partum depression in the US, but can suggest some very fruitful avenues for investigating the role of social support to new mothers.

There are two distinct forms of medicine-taking: adherent medicine-taking and self-regulation. The latter reflects aversion to medicines. The use of alternative coping strategies is one expression of this aversion. In self-regulation, patients carry out their own cost-benefit analyses, informed by their own cultural meanings and resources. . . .' (Britten et al. 2002: 5)

The process of analysis is, then, very similar to that of analysing primary data, in that published findings are compared, contrasted, and integrated into a coherent argument. Meta-ethnography offers a qualitative approach to utilizing published research reports through synthesizing findings on topics where there has already been a considerable number of good-quality published studies.

Methodological issues in using documentary sources

Using existing sources if possible is, we have argued, often an efficient approach to research and one that can be used to address a wide range of qualitatively different research questions. It is not, though, always the method of choice, and a number of potential limitations need to be considered. First, the researcher is limited to what is available and accessible. Pat Holden, whose study of nursing in Uganda was discussed above, could draw on papers kept by the Overseas Nursing Association, but not all organizations keep their records, or would allow a researcher access to them. Second, data collected or generated for one purpose (even for research purposes) might be difficult to use to answer a different research question. It can be difficult to know before becoming immersed in the data what kind of research questions they will answer. This is a particular problem when designing research studies that need a clear research question at the outset (see Chapter 2). Third, the researcher has no control over, or often much knowledge of, how the data were collected. These issues will be more or less constraining on the feasibility of a study, largely depending on the methodological perspective employed.

Methodological perspectives

The illustrations used so far suggest that documents (like any data) can be read in a number of ways, depending on the perspective of the researcher. Within a positivist framework, we can see documents as representing some reality about the world, whether that is health care policies represented in written policy documents, or mortality rates represented by government reports of them, or women's experiences of the post-partum period. The same documents can also be read as giving us insight into the perspectives of those who produced them. So letters to magazines, or diaries, or official reports are a source of information for interpretative researchers in exploring the world-views of those who produce documents.

Bridget O'Laughlin (1998) takes this perspective in her discussion of the analysis of *grey literature*: unpublished reports from governmental and non-governmental organizations. For O'Laughlin, grey literature is an important source of information not about the topic of the report, but about the political processes that produced it. Drawing on her experience of researching policy-orientated development issues, she argues that the report is 'the outcome of a process of negotiation between researchers and the commissioning institution' (1998: 107), and analysis of the document depends on locating it within the political processes and competing institutional discourses within which it was produced. To do this involves reading them with prior knowledge of the topic, and with a sensitivity to what has been omitted, what solutions are framed as possible, whose voices are present and absent, and what power relations exist between the subjects of the report, the writers and the commissioners. Grey literature is an essential clue in explorations of the political process:

> It tells us the ways in which important institutions in the politics of development, such as the World Bank, UNICEF, COSATU (the South African trade union federation) and national governments, view problems and solutions in the domain we are studying. When a poverty study on Mozambique informs us that the 'prospects for off-farm employment in Mozambique ... have never been very bright' (World Bank 1989) we learn that current World Bank thinking on Mozambique ignores the long history of migrant labour. ... (O'Laughlin 1998: 111)

For social constructionists, documents represent clues to the ways in which aspects of the world (diagnostic categories, management structures, policies) are socially produced. David Armstrong's (1986) work on infant mortality (Case Study 7.1, above) is one example. Another is Tom Shakespeare's (1999) analysis of medical and disability rights discourses in genetics. He explores the various narratives evident in public discourses about genetic technologies, identified by reviewing major journals and textbooks in the field. Medical writing about genetics, he argues, utilizes narratives of tragedy, in the metaphors about those with disabilities and the genes themselves (described as 'bad' or 'defective'), and of optimism in describing the potential role of medicine. Noting that the eugenic position is not presented in any clear-cut way in these accounts, he points to the methodological limitations of focusing purely on public documents as a source:

> ... [there is] a need to try and gather more unguarded statements or undertake qualitative research. Methodologically, this raises a problem for disabled researchers, because it

suggests that clinicians and researchers would present different accounts of their views to a disabled researcher than they might to someone seen as less implicated in the new technologies. (Shakespeare 1999: 672)

Despite pointing to these limitations of 'public' documents as a source, Shakespeare does demonstrate their utility. In analysing the contrasting rhetorics of medical writers and disability activists, he identifies what is missing in the debate: a nuanced, balanced account of the embodied experiences of people with disabilities, and the challenges faced in developing an understanding of the potential and dangers of genetic research.

Whatever the orientation of the researcher, we have suggested that using existing sources of data has many advantages, including efficiency and the ready availability of many sources. However, there are some drawbacks to using documents as primary data, whether from public records, personal documents, media output or research products. In positivist approaches, some key considerations include threats to reliability and validity.

Threats to reliability

One major concern with reliability is the representativeness of records. Two sources of bias operate to potentially limit representativeness. First is *selective deposit*; that is, that not everything gets recorded (or published, or photographed) at the time. A second source of bias is *selective survival*, in that what survives of any data set is not necessarily representative of what is deposited (Webb et al. 1977). In Oinas's study of letters to Finnish magazines, for instance, she notes that we cannot assume that those who write letters are in any way representative of the wider population of Finnish young women, or even that those letters that get published are representative of all those who write. These limitations would be important from a positivist perspective, if we were, for instance, attempting to review the evidence to identify exactly what young women's concerns about menstruation were, but Oinas's study is not attempting to answer this question. From a more positivist perspective, we can see how in Case Study 7.2 one particular cause of selective deposit, publication bias, might be more problematic. It may be that reports of post-partum symptoms in non-Western cultures are simply less likely to get reported. In this study, the authors have to consider how to guard against conclusions based on a potentially biased set of data. Threats to reliability are, then, an issue for some research questions, but in others are better thought of as limitations on the kinds of questions we can ask of any particular data set, rather than limitations in the data themselves.

Threats to validity

A basic issue of the validity of a document is its authenticity: is the document genuinely what it purports to be? This may be a particular problem with historical sources such as diaries or letters, which may be deliberate 'fakes', such as the 'Hitler Diaries', or produced as fiction intended to imitate personal record. Again, from a positivist perspective, threats to validity have to be carefully considered. In more interpretative traditions, however, 'truth' is rather more complex, as Norman Denzin suggests:

> The problem involves facts, facticities and fiction. *Facts* refer to events that are believed to have occurred or will occur. ... *Facticities* describe how those facts were lived and experienced by interacting individuals. ... *Fiction* is a narrative which deals with real or imagined facts and facticities. *Truth* refers ... to statements that are in agreement with facts and facticities as they are known and commonly understood. ... A truthful fiction (narrative) is faithful to facticities and facts. It creates verisimilitude, or what are for the reader believable experiences. (Denzin 1989a: 23)

For Denzin, then, the essential question of validity (is this a true account?) is a rather inadequate one when faced with biographical sources from an interpretative perspective, as we are treating the text as essentially a literary artefact, and the aim is understanding the subjective experience of an individual, not merely accruing 'facts' about their life. For qualitative approaches outside the positivist traditions, threats to reliability and validity may be less relevant, as the object of research is what has been preserved, or cited, or is available, and the questions asked of documents relate to the social reality they represent or shape, rather than reflect.

A broader methodological drawback is that documents alone may furnish few clues about their production. If we are interested, for instance, in a policy process, documents may tell us little about the decision-making that led to the policy, or the role of particular groups or individuals in its formation. In the study by Oinas of letters to magazines, described above, we know nothing about the motivations of the writers, how the letters were selected for publication or how they were edited by the magazine's staff. Of course, a research study can always include complementary components to address these questions of production, such as interviews with policy-makers or journalists, and in practice many projects will use a number of methodological strategies in tandem.

Conclusion

This chapter has highlighted the potential uses of documentary evidence for health research. The key advantages of documentary sources, especially for unfunded student projects, lie in their efficiency, in that many documents (such as published research reports, official statistics, newspaper articles and published biographical sources) are usually freely available from libraries, reasonably easily accessible, and it will take less time to assemble a data set than if producing primary data. Even data sources that take a little more effort (such as archived primary data, or mass media outputs) will require less time than field-work or a series of interviews. In addition to practical advantages, documents offer the potential for analysis from a number of qualitative perspectives. We have discussed in this chapter examples such as: positivist analysis of research outputs (Case Study 7.2); social constructionist analysis of public records (Case Study 7.1) and research outputs (Kaufert's study of papers on the menopause); interpretative studies of research outputs (Britten et al.'s meta-analysis of papers on medicine-taking); and critical approaches to grey literature (O'Laughlin's comments on reading reports from development institutions). But of course, this does not exhaust either the range of approaches or the potential sources that could be used. One source we haven't touched on, for instance, is arte-facts. Qualitative sociology is perhaps most associated with language data, whether oral or from texts, but it has been argued that this has marginalized other material sources of documentary evidence, particularly visual documents such as photographs and art, which could also offer much for qualitative research questions (Harrison 1996). Anthropology has perhaps a stronger tradi-tion of interest in the artefacts of material culture, but they are still perhaps underutilized as evidence on which we can draw in studies of health and related topics. The field of health has a rich material culture, including medical instruments, therapeutic and diagnostic artefacts, the material outcomes of therapy (such as x-rays, medical records), clothing (professional uniforms, safety wear), laboratory equipment and architecture, that has attracted some research, but is generally underdeveloped. Like any documents, or indeed any other data sources, these can be 'read' in a number of ways, depending on the orientations of the researcher and the research questions they are addressing.

KEY POINTS

- Using existing documents can be an efficient strategy for health research projects, usually requiring fewer resources than producing primary data.
- Accessible sources include public records, personal documents, mass media outputs, and research data and outputs.
- Documents can be analysed from a range of epistemological perspectives.

EXERCISES

1 Suggest some potential research studies you could carry out using health promotion posters in a health clinic as your data source. What could these posters tell you about:
   (a) The health problems considered important in this area?
   (b) How messages about these health problems are framed?
   What are the limits to posters as a data source to answer these ques-tions?

2 What other sources of documentary data could be used in a study of health promotion policy? For each you identify, consider the possible research questions you could address using this data source, and its limitations.

FURTHER READING

Plummer, K. (1983) *Documents of life: an introduction to the problems and literature of a humanistic method.* London: Unwin Hyman. Ken Plummer's text is a plea for the serious consideration of sources such as life histories in the social sciences, as a way of accessing subjective meanings and lived experiences. He introduces some of the classic literature, the history of the method and how to go about doing a life history.

8

Analysing Qualitative Data

CHAPTER SUMMARY

Analysis of qualitative data relies on both rigour and imagination. In health research, qualitative researchers are increasingly expected to report their methods of analysis in a transparent way. This chapter focuses on methods to improve rigour, and introduces three approaches to analysis common in health research (thematic content analysis, grounded theory, framework analysis). Strategies for improving the reliability and validity of analysis are discussed.

Approaches to analysis

In disciplines such as sociology and anthropology, there has traditionally been little emphasis on techniques for the analysis of qualitative data. Indeed, many of the classic studies that have had an impact on the health field have little information about how the data were analysed, and the most cited works tend to be predominantly theoretical, with few empirical findings (Chard et al. 1997). Even those based on empirical research, such as Goffman's *Asylums* (1961), on the social worlds of a mental hospital, rarely describe the *processes* of data analysis used. With the uptake of qualitative research designs in studies of health, rather than 'health' topics being coincidentally the subject of social science inquiry, and the growing market of peer-reviewed journals as outlets for qualitative research findings, there has been, though, a substantial increase in attention to the practice of analysis. This has addressed both the practical 'tools' or procedures researchers use to make sense of their data and the epistemological assumptions underpinning these techniques. In writing for audiences less familiar with social science writing, qualitative health researchers have had to be more explicit about what they *do* with data, and how their conclusions are built up from their interpretations. This has had benefits for relatively inexperienced researchers, who are often reassured by a set of steps that can be followed when faced with the task of making sense of data. It also, more arguably, has benefits for the non-social scientists who are the users of qualitative research in helping them judge whether the analysis was likely to have been done with due regard to issues of validity, rigour and comprehensiveness.

However, it is impossible to reduce the task of analysing qualitative data to a set of tools that can be applied in a mechanistic way. Good analysis (in quantitative as well as qualitative work) draws widely on more general social science knowledge, and locates the particular findings of one study within a broader context. The American sociologist C. Wright Mills described this as a 'sociological imagination' (Wright Mills 1959), an ability to 'shift from one perspective to another' (1959: 7), and to make the links between them. Thus it is rarely sufficient to focus purely on the data collected when doing analysis. Understanding the 'meaning' of data properly involves a broader perspective on history, social structures and comparative cases as well as an in-depth grasp of the particularities of the data set in question. To develop rules for integrating the more contextual and theoretical insights that contribute to analysing data is perhaps impossible: this constitutes the 'art' of qualitative analysis, utilizing imagination (the ability to make links) as well as a broad-ranging knowledge base to draw upon. Norman Denzin (1994) argues that this art can only be learned by doing, and by thinking about interpretation as a kind of storytelling, in which practising the various conventions used develops an imaginative and theoretical approach.

To make claims for the importance of this 'imagination' is not the same as claiming that qualitative analysis is merely 'made up', and that the meanings inherent in data can be whatever the analyst wants them to be. Qualitative analysis should be rigorous as well as imaginative, and the requirements of thoroughness, reliability and attention to validity provide a necessary, if not sufficient, condition for conducting good and useful work in health research. The interpretations made by the researcher have to be credible, and the links between the empirical data and the claims made about them clear. This chapter concentrates on techniques for maximizing rigour, because these are the bedrock of good analysis. Outlining guidelines for the creative aspects of analysis is more difficult. For many people, this is an intuitive skill, but it is one that can be developed with experience and the cultivation of an inquiring approach.

Styles of analysis

There is a broad range of approaches to analysis in qualitative research, with the task of the researcher defined rather differently across that range. In the more humanistic traditions, the researcher may be conceptualized more as a 'conduit', through which other voices can be heard, than an analyst. If the aims of the study are to give voice to participants, and represent their individual subjective experiences, then talking of 'analysis' is perhaps inappropriate, and the task of presenting the raw data to a wider audience may be more akin to editing than analysis. If the researcher's aim is to allow participants to 'speak for themselves', their analytical task may be minimal, restricted to merely tidying up sections of transcript for publication. Ken Plummer's approach to life histories perhaps epitomizes the humanist tradition, in that he talks about a continuum of researcher 'contamination' (Plummer 1983: 113). At one end of his continuum is theoretical analysis that has taken no account of subjective experience, where empirical data are not really used. At the other end is simple editing of life-history documents, where the researcher publishes accounts (from diaries, interviews or other sources) with no explicit interpretation, and the story is allowed to 'speak for itself'.

This chapter is concerned with the problem of studies in the middle of Plummer's continuum: those that utilize empirical data from the 'lifeworld' of everyday accounts, but that wish to go beyond merely reporting those accounts. Most approaches to analysing qualitative data attempt to 'intervene' at some level, to draw out the 'meaning' of the data that are not obvious at a journalistic or narrative reading. In health research, there are also usually requirements to be explicit about how the data were analysed, and how the 'stories' or other material are selected, interpreted and organized. Broadly, the aims of most qualitative analysis are to both reflect the complexity of the phenomena studied, and to present the underlying structures that 'make sense' of that complexity. The task of the researcher is thus a dual and perhaps inherently contradictory one of simultaneously 'telling the story' from the point of view of the research participants, and unpacking that story in some way such that the broader meanings can be elicited. One way in which styles of analysis can be distinguished is in terms of the extent to which they maintain the integrity of the data, in aiming to reproduce for the reader a contextual, in-depth picture of a social setting, life story or experience. Description is of course a basic building block of all analysis styles, but in some a more holistic description is more central than in others, which focus more on 'unpacking' the data to reveal the underlying patterns.

Relating analysis to the aims of the study

The approach adopted for managing and analysing data from an empirical study is of course related to the aims of the study. One influence on the kind of analysis used will be what the findings are intended to do, whether it is to contribute to sociological theory, evaluate a health promotion intervention or inform the development of a survey questionnaire. These broad aims will influence the *style* of analysis: whether it attempts to merely report the views of the respondents, or a more detailed analysis that aims to explain how the accounts produced in the research illuminate a particular research question. Some common approaches are outlined below, but at a general level, analysis might aim for some of the following outcomes:

- Developing conceptual definitions.
- Developing typologies and classifications.
- Exploring associations between attitudes, behaviours and experiences.
- Developing explanations of phenomena.
- Generating new ideas and theories.

If you look back at the study of asthma patients described in Case Study 1.1, some of these are illustrated. The researchers use a *conceptual definition* of 'stigma' that has been developed through other qualitative work (Goffman 1963) to look at responses to asthma. From their own data, the authors identify a *typology* of three broad responses to asthma diagnosis: denial, acceptance and pragmatism. Within the data, they look at how attitudes (to, for instance, what kind of disease asthma is) are *associated with* experiences and behaviours such as taking medication, using the asthma clinic and disclosing diagnosis to others. Finally, they were thus able to develop some *explanations* of phenomena such as the low 'compliance' with preventative medication.

Principles of different approaches

In practice, most researchers probably use a pragmatic mixture of approaches to analysis within any particular study. The approaches taken may not be cited explicitly in written reports, especially if writing for a social science rather than a health audience. Those selected reflect both the needs of a particular project and the epistemological assumptions the researcher makes about what the data can tell them. Here, we outline three common approaches: thematic content analysis, grounded theory and framework analysis. These have all been widely used in health research, and the differences between them illustrate the differences in emphasis across the range of qualitative research.

Thematic content analysis

The most basic type of qualitative analysis is an analysis of the content of the data to categorize the recurrent or common 'themes'. This is perhaps the most common approach used in qualitative research reported in health journals, and aims to report the key elements of respondents' accounts. It is a useful approach for answering questions about the salient issues for particular groups of respondents or identifying typical responses. In a study of community views about health needs, for instance, identifying the main themes in interviewees' accounts might be the main aim of the study.

Using data such as interview notes or transcripts, the researcher looks through them to categorize respondents' accounts in ways that can be summarized. It is essentially a comparative process, by which the various accounts gathered are compared with each other to classify those 'themes' that recur or are common in the data set. The easiest way to do this kind of analysis is using 'scissors and paste'. In the margins of each transcript or set of notes, go through to mark up the content of what is being said by labelling excerpts. Box 8.1 shows an example of a section of transcript marked up for some of the key themes. This is an extract from a focus group interview with people with glaucoma, and the aims of the analysis here were to look for triggers to referral and to describe the problems faced by people with these kinds of eyesight problems. (There is more detail on the study from which this was taken in Case Study 8.1, below.)

There are a number of ways of laying out interview transcripts, but it is important to have some consistent format that leaves enough room for notes on the printed version. The extract in Box 8.1 illustrates some useful conventions: each new speaker starts on a new line, line numbers are used to make the extracts easier to reference, and short lines leave margins wide enough for coding. Note how codes might overlap: in lines 19–22, Donna's account of 'coping on her own' could be labelled as an example of both 'problems' faced, and as an example of 'strategies to cope' ('sister helping', using a white stick). For more detailed coding, it would be preferable to leave more space than in this extract.

Coding schemes (a list of code names to apply to the data) can be developed by looking through the early data to identify the key themes and how they will be labelled (the 'code'). If you are working as part of a team, you will need to discuss and agree on what the evidence for themes and codes is (that is, how particular utterances are 'indicators' of the concepts of interest) with your colleagues. If working alone, it is productive to consult with colleagues or a supervisor if possible during the early stages of data analysis. For instance, in Box 8.1, the extract starts with Ann's line 'we all look normal' (line 1) and

---

Box 8.1   Extract from focus group with five women with glaucoma, with themes marked

1. **Ann:** The problem is that we all look, well, normal. It's not like	Symbols of
2. we're carrying white sticks or anything –	disability/passing
3. **Bertha:** No, and even if you're being guided, you could just be	Passing
4. with a friend or something	
5. **Connie:** I've got a white stick – but usually it's in my handbag!	
6. I hate using it – people stare at you, and you get offered seats on	Stigma
7. the bus – you get more attention, more than I want anyway	
8. **Ann:** Well, that's the problem – it's embarrassing. People,	Misunderstandings
9. people, who don't know, assume	
10. that if you're using a white stick, you can't see anything, so	
11. they look – quite openly, staring, thinking you can't see them	Embarrassment
12. staring.	
13. **Interviewer:** So do you prefer looking 'normal'?	
14. **Bertha:** Well, I feel pretty normal, mostly	
15. **Connie:** With the white stick – it's meant for car drivers, really,	Aids for coping
16. so they see you in case you suddenly jump in the road – but I	
17. do feel very conscious when I'm carrying it. People jump out	
18. of the way like you've got the plague or something.	Stigma
19. **Donna:** I use one when I'm out on my own, when my sister's	
20. not with me, and it's mainly for dealing with stairs – I have	Aids for coping
21. problems with steps, not being able to see, with depth	Problems
22. perception –	
23. **Ann:** Oh, me too!	
24. **Donna:** – and contrasts, you know, coming into a dark room	Problems
25. outside, can't see a thing	Impact of problems
26. **Bertha:** Oh, god, lifts are the worst! I just can't see anything	
27. when I step into a lift –	
28. **Connie:** because it's all dark! I know – you just have to hope	Strategies for
29. someone else comes in to press the buttons	coping
30. **Ann:** That's why I wear dark glasses outside – it makes the	Strategies for
31. contrast less	coping

Bertha's response (lines 3–4) about being with a guide looking like being with a friend. In discussion, it was agreed that these were examples of 'looking normal' as opposed to 'disabled'. This was in contrast to when they were carrying white sticks, when people could identify them as 'disabled'. We therefore labelled this code as 'Passing', to summarize a key theme: ways in which participants thought they looked 'normal' in everyday life. In qualitative work, it is more common to develop the coding scheme from the empirical data, but elements of it may be predetermined by the research questions. In the example in Case Study 8.1, one aim of the study was to look at 'triggers for referral' – the signs and symptoms that people noticed, and that prompted them to seek help. This was therefore one element of the coding scheme, with a heading of 'Triggers for referral', although others were added as the data were analysed.

Copies of transcripts or notes can then literally be cut up and rearranged in piles or on large sheets of paper under the headings of the themes. In their focus group guidebook, Krueger and Casey (2000: 132–5) describe some practical suggestions for the 'scissor and paste' method of analysis:

- use a long table (or walls, or floor) covered with flip chart or newspaper, with sections headed with themes (or interview questions);
- distinguish each of one set of transcript copies by printing each on different coloured paper, or using coloured lines down the margins so that the original source of extracts cut out can be identified;
- cut the transcripts up into separate extracts;
- begin sorting extracts by assigning them to sections, and then comparing each new extract one with the growing pile: is it similar, or should you start a new pile or section?

These kinds of cut and paste techniques are 'low technology', but they work. They allow the researcher, or team of researchers, to compare, contrast, start to build up categories and typologies and to discuss the 'meaning' of their data. Word processors have made these processes a little easier, in that you can cut and paste transcripts on screen into new documents, with a separate document for each emerging theme. If there are a small number of interview transcripts, each can be identified with a different font, or colour. With larger data sets, you may have to type in a case identifier for the original transcript after each quote. At this point, the advantages of using computer software to help with the analysis start emerging (see below).

This kind of thematic analysis can be as simple or sophisticated as is needed for the project in hand. If doing exploratory work in an area where not much is known, it may be enough to simply report the common issues mentioned in a community, and go no further than listing each issue, perhaps with some quoted excerpts to give 'colour'. If the qualitative study is a pilot for developing a questionnaire, you may want to pay more attention to how respondents discussed particular issues: what terminology they used, how difficult it was to talk about, and how often particular issues were mentioned.

Thematic analysis is also the basis of more sophisticated qualitative analysis, in which the researcher moves beyond simply categorizing and coding the data to thinking about how the codes relate to each other and asking more complex questions. The example in Box 8.1, for instance, shows the 'first level' of thematic analysis of some focus group data. One outcome of this could be 'lists' of issues, such as a list of common problems faced by people with glaucoma in work, family life and leisure activities and a list of initial symptoms that alerted people to their eye problems. One of the aims of the study from which this is taken was to inform health promotion activities for encouraging people to attend for eye tests, and this basic level of analysis is perhaps sufficient for this, as it provides some information from respondents about the kinds of information likely to be useful to the target population. However, to take this further, we might want to look at *relationships* between the themes that emerged, and look at the context of particular codes. Questions an analyst could ask to facilitate this might include:

- Which kinds of respondents are more likely to report problems of daily living? Men, women, those who were relatively young when their glaucoma was diagnosed, those with little family support?
- Which kinds of respondents are more likely to report feelings of stigma, and is this related to their views of eye problems?
- How do respondents' accounts of their diagnosis relate to their accounts of current problems?

Thematic analysis is, then, enough for many health research projects, particularly if they are exploratory or the aim is to describe the key issues of concern to a particular group of people. However, many qualitative researchers will want to ask rather more of their data, and other techniques are needed if we are to move beyond the 'emic' summaries and typologies of participants' accounts that a thematic analysis provides. A good qualitative analysis should also say something about social life, as well as what participants say about it. It should provide a 'thick', rich description of the setting studied, link into theory, and provide a satisfying and credible account of 'what is going on'. Two potential ways of developing a deeper analysis of qualitative data are grounded theory (sometimes called the constant comparative method) and framework analysis. They share many features, but are rather different in emphasis, so we describe them here separately.

Grounded theory

One approach to taking a more systematic view of qualitative data analysis was developed by two American sociologists, Barney Glaser and Anslem Strauss (Glaser and Strauss 1967; Strauss 1987). Their writings on what they called 'grounded theory' have been extremely influential on qualitative research. Glaser and Strauss attempted to operationalize the procedures they thought informed much qualitative analysis, but which were never written down. They argued that you could unpack the rules researchers use to, as they put it, 'discover theory from data' and that, with practice, most people could learn to use them. So it was in some ways an attempt to demystify the processes of qualitative analysis, and to provide a set of what they called 'rules of thumb' to help develop theory that was grounded in empirical data. Although this suggests an inductive method of research, in which theory is built up from empirical observations (rather than deductive, in which theories are 'tested' against the data), Glaser and Strauss argue that the strength of grounded theory approaches lies in the cyclical process of collecting data, analysing it, developing a provisional coding scheme, using this to suggest further sampling, more analysis, checking out emerging theory, and so on, until a point of 'saturation' is reached, when no new constructs are emerging. At this point, you have a rich, dense theoretical account – but one that is completely grounded in empirical data. It is thus both inductive and deductive, moving back and forward between emerging theory and data. The other key principle (and why this is also known as the 'constant comparative method') is 'constant comparison', and the notion that interpretation of data moves forward through comparing indicators (codes), cases and data sets.

A first step in a grounded theory analysis is the emphasis on intense coding of early data. This entails *open coding*, an intense line-by-line analysis of, say, a transcript, that attempts to open up or 'fracture' the data. This forces you to take a step back and open up all potential avenues of inquiry. In taking a small part of early data phrase by phrase, and asking the general question 'what's going on here?', the idea is to generate as many potential codes as possible. It doesn't matter if these are 'wrong' at this stage, as grounded theory involves going back to the data to check these emerging ideas, and refining the concepts and 'theories' about them throughout the research process. By 'codes' Glaser and Strauss do not mean merely descriptive summaries of the data, but more conceptual labels, which identify what general phenomenon is indicted by the instance, or extract of talk, being analysed.

To take an example from Box 8.1, we might start with lines 1–4, and interrogate these for the possible answers to 'what is going on here?' Some potential questions one might ask of these data are: How does Ann constitute 'looking normal'? Why does she say this is a problem? What signs of 'normality' are there in everyday appearances? Why would a white stick undermine this appearance of normality? Why would being guided undermine an appearance of normality? How is being guided different from being with a friend? Asking this barrage of questions intensively around a few lines of data helps generate some useful early ideas about the data, and lines of inquiry to follow. Even from these few lines, we might develop some initial concepts, including:

Constituting normality (how people behave normally, how they assess it in others)
Constituting disability (how disability is communicated)

Each of these initial concepts is subjected to further questions, in order to explore its *properties* and its *dimensions*. Properties are attributes, or characteristics. In the example above, the properties of 'constituting disability' might include behaving in remarkable ways, looking unusual, using mobility aids. Dimensions are the continua along which these properties can be arranged. For instance, one concept in the study of glaucoma was 'onset of sight problems'. The dimensions of this include: rate of onset (sudden, gradual) and expectedness (expected, unexpected). Open coding can quickly generate a long list of concepts, which can then be categorized into a more sophisticated scheme by gathering together those that appear to relate to similar phenomena.

One set of codes to look for are what Glaser and Strauss call *in vivo codes* – the kinds that participants use themselves to divide up the world. In the short extract in Box 8.1, there are a number of in vivo codes suggested. The idea of 'looking normal' is one, and we could look through the transcripts to look for what it categorizes: what examples are given of people who don't 'look normal'? Another is at lines 8–9, of 'people who don't know', which could be contrasted with 'sister', and perhaps other examples of 'people who do know' in the transcripts. Examples of in vivo codes can be found in most data, and are useful first steps in exploring how respondents see their social worlds. A common one in many medical settings is the way in which professionals classify their patients or clients into categories such as 'good patients', 'interesting patients' and other, less complimentary, categories. One example is from Roger Jeffrey's (1979) study of 'normal rubbish' as an in vivo category used by staff in an Accident and Emergency department to describe the patients they did not find interesting or deserving. These in vivo codes are useful as first steps in categorizing the data, though the analysis has to go further than simply noting them. In Jeffrey's study, he unpicked the criteria by which staff categorized patients, and linked these to normative ideas about legitimacy in sickness.

All codes should be labelled, at least provisionally, as the process of naming them is part of the work of thinking about what they are: What is the concept that this particular code relates to? What connects the different instances (extracts) that are coded in this way? This helps moves the analysis from a rather descriptive level, where the researcher is merely summarizing what is in the data, to a more analytical level, which is focused on the phenomena in the data as examples of some more generalizable concepts.

Initial open coding is a first step, but can be returned to at any point when the data analysis becomes 'stuck'. However, it is obviously too intensive to apply to the whole data set. Once a provisional coding scheme has been developed, the analysis can move to the next stage, *axial coding*, in which the fractured data are 'put back together again'. Here, the analysis moves on to looking for relationships between categories. For the glaucoma study example, this might include looking at the following questions: How does suddenness of onset of symptoms relate to problems of daily living? Is there a relationship between 'passing' as normal and attitudes to eye disease? One strategy for axial coding is developing a coding paradigm, which entails a set of questions about each code. These are: What conditions give rise to the category? What is its context? What are the interactional strategies by which it is handled and what are the consequences of those strategies? For example, for the category 'passing as normal', we might therefore develop the following:

Conditions: feeling that 'blindness' is stigmatizing
Context: being in public, being with strangers
Interactional strategies: not using white sticks, not going out alone
Consequences: strain of managing, embarrassment

Finally, more *selective coding*, where the aim is to move towards more abstract and analytical and theoretically informed concepts, is the stage at which the core categories emerge. These are essential in that they are related to most other categories, and explain most of what is going on.

Because grounded theory moves from inductive to deductive modes, and back and forward between theory and data, it ideally relies on what Glaser and Strauss call 'theoretical sampling'. The cases to include should be dictated by the emerging data, and data analysis will suggest further cases to investigate. In addition to advocating that data collection and analysis continue simultaneously, rather than sequentially, grounded theory also involves writing throughout the process. These ongoing written records are called 'memos', defined as 'the written forms of our abstract thinking about the data' (Strauss and Corbin 1990: 198). Writing memos is an essential part of the analysis, rather than something begun towards the end of a project. Memos will include operational notes about data collection, but also theoretical memos, which are an essential step in the development of analytical ideas. Theoretical memos include initial ideas about the data, emerging hypotheses about relationships between codes and the properties of codes, and detailed notes later in the analysis on how the axial and selective coding is developing.

Kathy Charmaz, discussing the importance of memos in her work (Charmaz 1999), describes them as a 'pivotal intermediate step between coding and writing', which allow the researcher to stop and think about the data and move beyond descriptive 'codes' to thinking about how codes can become categories for analysis, and alerting the researcher to gaps in the data and points where comparisons can be made. Crucially, she suggests, memos keep the researcher writing, which is an essential element in the analysis itself (see Chapter 10).

Key to analysis in grounded theory is the constant attempt to challenge and develop theoretical insights. A close attention to *deviant cases* is crucial to this, in which the researcher both deliberately, through theoretical sampling, includes data with which to test the emerging theory, and pays close attention to the exceptions within the data set. The two case studies in this chapter have examples of the use of deviant cases.

Finally, it should be noted that 'grounded theory' is perhaps one of the most abused phrases in the qualitative health literature. Increasingly, researchers are making claims to have used a 'grounded theory' approach in what emerges as rather superficial thematic content analysis. An analysis that has used grounded theory should provide a detailed, saturated account of the data, rather than a list of 'key themes'. It should be possible to read the account to see how variation within the data set has been used comparatively to develop the analysis, and how deviant cases have contributed to a credible and thorough account of the data.

To do 'grounded theory', and reach this point of theoretical saturation, is time-consuming, and much health research is constrained by practical issues of policy and funding. One constraint is on the flexibility sponsors will allow in collecting more data, or different data, as a result of early analysis. A second is of course time scale. Most projects are done to tight deadlines, and it is doubtful how often this saturation really happens. Nonetheless, the principles and some of the approaches of grounded theory have been invaluable to health research-ers, and even if funding and resources do not allow the researchers to develop a saturated grounded theory, there are many elements of the grounded theory approach that are useful for any analysis. Open coding, for instance, can be an insightful way of bringing fresh ideas to your analysis, and ensuring that you have developed some 'analytical distance'. Case Study 8.1 used elements of the grounded theory approach to analyse data.

Framework analysis

The stated aim of grounded theory is development of theory. Obviously this will throw up policy-relevant findings, and much of the work in this tradition has developed our understanding of health and health services in ways that have quite profound implications for practice. However, the aim of policy devel-opment is not at the forefront, and generally grounded theory, given that we can't say at the beginning what we will find out, or even who we are going to include in the sample, is not easy to sell to policy- and practice-minded fun-ders. Framework analysis, on the other hand, developed by the National Centre for Social Research (http://www.scpr.ac.uk/), is explicitly geared towards generating policy- and practice-orientated findings, and is popular with many health and social researchers for this reason (Ritchie and Spencer 1994). Described by the National Centre for Social Research as 'a content analysis method which involves summarising and classifying data within a the-matic framework', the key difference between this and 'grounded theory' approaches is that the integrity of individual respondents' accounts is preserved throughout the analysis, rather than the deliberate attempt to 'fracture' the data in order to open up new avenues for analysis.

Reflecting this focus on maintaining the integrity of respondents' narratives, the first step in framework analysis is *familiarization* with the data. This involves listening to tapes and re-reading fieldnotes or transcripts until the researcher is closely familiar with them in their entirety. Following on, the second step is a *thematic analysis* to develop a coding scheme. The themes in the data become the labels for codes. In framework analysis, the process of applying codes to the whole data set in a systematic way is called *indexing*. Indexing is the third step. Like grounded theory, the analysis part of framework analysis entails compar-ison, both within and between cases. This is facilitated by the fourth step, called *charting*, which involves rearranging the data according to this thematic content, either case by case, or by theme. These charts contain only summaries of data, so the researcher can see across cases and under themes the range of data. Summary examples in the charts are referenced back to the original transcript. Case Study 8.2 includes an extract of a chart from a study by Geraldine Barrett

Case Study 8.1   Using elements of the constant comparative method in a study of living with glaucoma

(Source: Green, J., Siddall, H. and Murdoch, I. (2002) 'Learning to live with glaucoma: a qualitative study of diagnosis and the impact of sight loss', *Social Science and Medicine*, 55: 257–67)

This study used individual and group interviews to explore the experiences of people who had been diagnosed with glaucoma, an eye disease characterized by gradual loss of visual acuity. The aims were to inform health promotion by identifying triggers and barriers to self-referral with eye problems, and to explore the relationship between 'medical' definitions of disability and people's experiences of sight problems.

Interviews took a narrative approach, asking interviewees to tell the story of how they first noticed eye problems, how they came to be referred for treatment, and what impact symptoms and treatment regimes had on their everyday lives. Interviews were tape-recorded and transcribed, and some participants also provided written notes on their experiences. Although this was not a 'grounded theory' study, some of the elements of the grounded theory approach were used to aid data analysis. One was the use of 'open coding' of early data to generate categories. This enabled the range of concepts used by participants to be identified, and to extend the analysis so that the research question could be better understood in terms of 'grounded' theory; that is, ideas from the data themselves. For instance, one research aim was to identify 'triggers for self-referral'. Although the data could be 'coded' for triggers (such as noticing blurred vision, noticing 'missing' patches in the field of vision), detailed analysis of the data, and of the contexts of these reported symptoms, suggested that these were 'post hoc' descriptions of triggers, and at the time the early 'signs' of glaucoma are indistinguishable from the everyday eye problems many expect as a result of tiredness or ageing.

A second element of grounded theory used was theoretical sampling. One emerging theory in the data analysis was that a worry about 'dependence' was a concern for some in the sample, but did not seem to be an issue for an older married man, who relied on his wife for extensive help in everyday tasks anyway. We then deliberately sampled older patients, and looked in detail at cases with a range of family support, to check emerging relationships between family support and concepts of dependence and independence.

Close attention to deviant cases helped develop the analysis. One example was the findings on attitudes to blindness. The majority of participants utilized one of two images of 'blind people': either the 'victim' who was to be pitied, because they were dependent on others, or the 'hero', who manages to perform extraordinary feats despite their disability. Not surprisingly, neither was a very appealing image, and most respondents did not identify themselves as 'blind'. Although (for them) this brought benefits such as passing as normal, and resisting the felt stigma of being labelled as blind, it had considerable costs as a strategy. For some, it meant they had no access to material benefits to which they were entitled. A 'deviant case' was one

man who had a less 'stigmatized' image of what blindness meant. He had
diabetes, and, because he already had come to terms with an identity
including 'disease', could see that 'being blind' did not have to be incompa-
tible with 'leading a normal life'.

Locating the empirical findings from this study within wider theoretical literature on disability and living with chronic illness helped make sense of
the data. There is a large literature on issues such as 'independence' and
'stigma', and this was used to help make sense of the accounts of people
with glaucoma.

The constant comparative approach, then, helped develop initial categories for coding, helped inform sampling, and provided a framework for
looking at relationships between categories.

and Kaye Wellings on how women use and define terms such as 'unplanned'
when talking about pregnancy. Note how this organizes data under themes for
each interviewee, and is annotated with page references to the interview
transcript, so that the original data can quickly be retrieved. These charts can
then be used to compare across each code, and see the whole range of phenomena, where they do and don't occur, and start to look at relationships
between codes.

What moves framework analysis beyond a sophisticated thematic analysis is
the final stage of looking at relationships between the codes. This is what is
known as *mapping and interpretation*, so a key tactic is to use diagrams and tables
to physically explore the relationships between the concepts and typologies
developed from them, and associations between the concepts. In Case Study
8.2, Barrett and Wellings are able to explore the use of different terms within
their sample, and look at the relationships between characteristics such as
contraceptive use and how pregnancy is discussed. Framework analysis in
general has an overt policy orientation, with an end point of developing
practical strategies on the basis of analysis. In this case study, the qualitative
study is used to inform the design of a survey, through the development of a
valid measure of pregnancy intention.

Using computer software to help manage data

Whatever approach, or mixture of approaches, is used, analysis requires considerable work, both mundane (coding data) and more creative (thinking about
categories). This can be very time-consuming. We have already mentioned
that word processors have made some tasks more efficient. The ability to 'cut
and paste' electronically between documents, insert automatic line numbering
and search for words or phrases are tasks that most word processors can do.
There are also, though, a number of dedicated software packages designed to

Case Study 8.2   An example of framework analysis from a study of how women discuss pregnancy planning and intention

(Sources: (1) Barrett, G. and Wellings, K. (2002) 'What is a "planned" pregnancy? Empirical data from a British study', *Social Science and Medicine*, 55: 545–57. (2) Barrett, G., Personal communication)

In the family-planning literature, terms such as 'planned/unplanned', 'intended/unintended' and 'wanted/unwanted' to describe pregnancy are often used as if their meaning was obvious and unproblematic, but there has been little research on how women themselves understand them. Geraldine Barrett and Kaye Wellings aimed to develop a valid measure of pregnancy planning/intention for use in quantitative surveys. A first step was a qualitative study with pregnant women that used in-depth interviews to collect data on a series of topics, including when they became aware that they were pregnant, their contraceptive use, feelings about being pregnant and decisions about the pregnancy. At the end of the interview, women were asked about their understanding of the terms planned, unplanned, intended, unintended, wanted and unwanted, and whether any of these terms applied to their own pregnancies.

When data collection was complete, framework analysis was used to analyse the data. The first four steps (familiarization, identifying a thematic framework and coding frame, indexing and charting) are described primarily as ways of managing the data. The table on page 188 shows this fourth stage of charting, in an extract from one of the charts.

Charting involves rearranging the data within themes so that it can be compared across the interviews and within each interview. Barrett and Wellings describe the fifth step, mapping and interpretation, as the crucial one in developing their analysis of the data, involving 'Drawing diagrams to clarify ideas . . . looking for associations between the concepts and women's characteristics (e.g. age, marital/partnership status), and discussing the meanings of what we found' (Barrett and Wellings 2002: 547).

Framework analysis provided an appropriate approach in a study where some of the research questions were predetermined. Thus, in order to explore whether women did or did not use particular terms spontaneously, how these compared with definitions that were prompted, and how the use of terms varied across the sample, it was helpful to arrange the data across charts by themes. Diagrams were a useful way of graphically illustrating findings, for instance by drawing circles of various sizes to illustrate how many women used particular definitions. By looking across the interviews, they are able to show the criteria by which women judge a pregnancy to be, for instance, 'planned' or 'unintended'.

Barrett and Wellings use a number of strategies to increase the credibility of their findings and the reliability and validity of the analysis. First, quotes from the interview transcripts are used as examples of particular definitions, so the reader can see how the interpretation is built on the data. There is enough detail (such as point in the interview) to judge the context of women's accounts. Second, they use numerical counts (of, for instance, how many women in the sample applied particular terms to their own preg-

Extract from chart produced for 'What is a planned pregnancy?' study

Interview No.	Partner's feelings about outcome	Partner's feelings about fatherhood	Definitions of planned/unplanned (introduced terms)	Definitions of intended/unintended (introduced terms)
105	Happy	Assumed would be father in future p. 8. Enjoys fatherhood p. 9	Planned – planned to have child p. 10. Unplanned is an accident p. 10	Intended – you intend to have the child, you wanted one p. 10. Unintended – not planning to have a child and finding they are pregnant p. 10, also accident
106	Happy	Says he probably wanted to be a father sooner than she wanted to be a mother p. 11. Very positive about fatherhood p. 11	Planned – same as intended pregnancy. Unplanned – not necessarily using contraception, had sex without contraception p. 13	Intended – actively set out to create child, not using contraception, using fertile period etc. p. 13. Unintended – not intending to get pregnant, either using contraception or just get pregnant by mistake p. 13 – moves towards seeing unintended as contraceptive failure p. 13
107	Nervous p. 4. Says he'll be at the birth p. 13	Says he never actually wanted to have children, nervous about being a bad father p. 12. He's acting as a father to her first child at the moment p. 12	Planned – trying for a baby, find out best time to fall pregnant. Unplanned – fall pregnant without meaning to p. 13	Intended and unintended – interchangeable with planned and unplanned p. 13
108	Happy	Doesn't think he always wanted to be a father – wanted to find right partner, could have considered life without children p. 12. Very happy as a father now p. 12	Planned – something you want very much, you try and create it p. 13. Planned and unplanned are similar to intended and unintended, but sound a bit more structured p. 16, more focused p. 17	Unintended – an accident, you didn't want or didn't consciously want. Intended – like planned p. 16
109	Nervous about birth p. 18	Doesn't really think of himself as a father yet p. 13	Planned and unplanned – like intended and unintended p. 20	Intended – you've planned for, actively tried to become pregnant. Unintended – pregnancy you weren't planning to have p. 19 – doesn't include not using contraception p. 20 (those are intended)

nancies). Third, they report 'deviant cases' and demonstrate how they can be accounted for within their explanations of the data. For instance, the majority of women who applied both the terms 'unplanned' or 'unintended' to their pregnancies reported (not surprisingly) in their interviews that they had neither planned nor intended their pregnancy. One exception is discussed in detail: a woman who reports that she had intended to become pregnant, but that the pregnancy itself was unplanned. Looking through the whole transcript, it was possible to see that this woman did not meet the criteria other women used to describe a pregnancy as 'planned'. Although, like most, she and her partner had agreed to try to conceive, and she had deliberately stopped taking contraception, unlike others who used both the terms 'unplanned' and 'unintended', they had not made wider preparations for a birth.

In summary, one key finding was the way in which the term 'planned' was used. Merely to have *intended* to become pregnant and stopped using contraception was not sufficient; women also used two other criteria: agreeing this decision with a partner, and making wider life preparations for a pregnancy. This suggests that a survey question such as 'Was your pregnancy planned?' might only elicit a positive response from those who met all four criteria, and many women who 'wanted' and 'intended' the pregnancy might not answer 'yes', if they did not also meet the conditions of agreement with partner and preparation.

---

help manage, and to some extent aid analysis of, qualitative data in more sophisticated ways. They include ETHNOGRAPH, ATLAS/ti, QSR NUD★IST and NVivo. These are currently the most widely used software packages. They have been developed by social researchers trying to meet their own needs and each has slightly different features that reflect their developer's outlook. NVivo is the most recently developed (this is another QSR package, slightly different from, but also acting as an upgrade to, NUD★IST 6) and the choice of name belies its conceptual approach. Its website describes it as:

a very richly featured and highly advanced program for handling Qualitative Data Analysis research projects. ... Researchers can handle rich data as rich text, using bold, italics, colours and other formatting – with full ability to edit, visually code and link documents as they are created, coded, filtered, managed and searched.

The QSR packages are probably the best supported, with up–to–date, easily accessible websites, dedicated e-mail lists and discussion fora. There are also several books and manuals to support NUD★IST and NVivo, with the most recent being *Using NVivo in Qualitative Research* (1999) by Lynn Richards (one of the developers), published by Sage. ATLAS/ti, on the other hand, is a somewhat smaller and altogether less 'corporate' affair, with a less hierarchical approach to data management. Both packages, however, retain strong links with their developers and both are published and distributed through Sage/ Scolari (the software publishing branch of Sage).

The first thing to stress is that none of these packages will do your analysis for you. They will help you to manage and retrieve data in more or less sophisticated ways, but the user still has to do the difficult tasks of developing a coding scheme, and coding the data. Both of these procedures can take longer if you are using a software package. Second, most packages have specific requirements for documents, and it is not always possible to directly import word processor files. If you are planning to use a particular package, try it out at the beginning of the project to make sure you produce the data (fieldnotes, or transcripts) in a compatible format. Formatting issues you may need to consider are: line length, line breaks between speakers or paragraphs, using consistent speaker identifiers, and the use of upper case. Third, if your analysis will be reliant on looking at the minutiae of interaction, such as the pauses, stresses and tone of everyday talk, most packages will not be able to handle the transcribing requirements of conversation analysis. Formatting such as underlining or bold is often eliminated, and packages may require punctuation such as full stops to mark section breaks.

The key advantage of using dedicated software packages is that the analysis can be more thorough and systematic than that done by hand. If the whole data set has been coded, searches for segments relating to codes will produce all relevant data, rather than just those excerpts that the researcher has noticed. On large or multi-site projects, using software can facilitate the transfer of data files, emerging coding schemes and research memos. This allows the whole team to contribute to analysis more easily, and has a secondary advantage of forcing greater transparency, as there is a record of how coding schemes were developed and theoretical concepts emerged through recorded memos. Some more sophisticated packages (such as ATLAS/ti) also provide 'added features', including the ability to handle graphics in the form of pictures that can be scanned in, and more complex ways of handling and mapping conceptual diagrams illustrating the relationships between codes.

Available packages and their capabilities change so rapidly that individual descriptions would quickly date, and it is advisable to use Internet sites to access details about available software. One useful source of information on software is the Computer Assisted Qualitative Data Analysis Software (CAQDAS) networking project website at http://www.soc.surrey.ac.uk/caqdas. This has links to demonstration versions of some of the packages, up-to-date guidelines for transcribing, a bibliography, and links to discussion groups. In general, though, Nigel Fielding (1994) describes packages as being of three main types:

- Those that retrieve particular kinds of text, such as searching for particular words or strings. These are useful for content analysis.
- Those that retrieve bits of text that you have coded, such as ETHNOGRAPH. These take over some of the 'cutting and pasting' work of collecting together instances of particular codes.

- Those that are designed with a particular theoretical approach – e.g. NUD★IST and ATLAS/ti – which allows you to build links between codes.

Some of the things you may want to consider when choosing a package are whether the program allows you to code directly on the screen, how much work it will take to prepare transcripts in a way that will work with the program, whether you can attach multiple codes to the same piece or overlapping pieces of text, whether you can include annotations or hyperlinks to your data, and how the results of your searches are displayed (Fielding 1995).

In summary, computer packages do not 'do analysis', but they can help both manage data and allow you to retrieve data quickly. This can help facilitate rigorous, thorough analysis. They are particularly useful if you have a large amount of data to manage, and also perhaps if you are working with a team of people who will need to use the data set and need a high level of transparency about coding frames and the process of analysis.

Rigour in analysis

The different styles of analysis outlined above emphasize different elements of the process, but there are a number of general principles that apply to most qualitative research. These are the kinds of 'good practice' guidelines that add credibility to your analysis, and increase faith in its reliability and validity. The criteria that typify rigorous analysis are summarized in Box 8.2.

Box 8.2 Some features of rigorous qualitative analysis

Criteria	Possible methods
Transparent	Provide a clear account of procedures used An 'audit trail' that others could follow
Maximizes validity	Analysis of deviant cases and disconfirming data 'Member validation' Including enough context for reader to judge interpretation
Maximizes reliability	Analysis of the whole data set Using more than one analyst/coder Simple frequency counts of key themes
Comparative	Compares data between and within cases in the data set Compares findings to other studies
Reflexive	Accounts for the role of the researcher in the research

Transparency

Transparency relates to the explicitness of the methods used, and how clearly they are outlined for the reader in research reports. This is perhaps a particularly important criterion when writing for audiences who may be unused to qualitative methods, such as biomedical journal readerships, or colleagues from other disciplines. The key is to provide an honest and clear account of the actual procedures used for analysing the data, rather than attempting to impress with jargon such as 'used a grounded theory approach' if this wasn't used. This might include a short description of how coding categories were developed, with perhaps examples of how debates around concepts led to labels for codes, how the sample was chosen (e.g. purposive sample? theoretical sample?), and how extracts used in the report were selected.

Maximizes validity

The validity of an interpretation is the 'truth' of that interpretation. In qualitative work, the notion of validity can be problematic, as in the interpretative and constructionist traditions we are working with 'truths' that are socially situated, and rejecting a positivist idea of one fixed and essential truth. However, this does not mean that qualitative researchers can dispense with all considerations of validity. There may be multiple readings of any particular data set, but the researcher does have to justify why their particular analysis should be considered a credible and legitimate one. Attempts to maximize validity are a way of answering the reader who asks 'Why should I believe this?' and 'How do I know this isn't just the researcher's subjective interpretation?' One common charge against qualitative work is anecdotalism – the idea that the researcher has merely reported anecdotes from the field that have struck a chord in some way but that are not rigorously and systematically supported by analysis. A similar charge is that of exoticism, with the suggestion that only the 'juicy quotes' or the most interesting or outlandish examples have been reported. In some of the social science traditions, presenting a subjective interpretation would be a legitimate exercise, but when working in health, especially if the research is aiming to influence policy or practice, it is usually necessary to demonstrate that the interpretation does have some validity: that the researcher has not focused only on the exotic, or drawn exclusively from the data that confirm their presumptions.

There are a number of approaches to increasing faith in validity. The key one is an approach that deliberately attempts to 'test' emerging theory. The aim should be to look for disconfirming evidence (such as deviant cases) and account for them, rather than just trawling through the data for examples that illustrate the points you want to make.

Simple counts can increase the reader's faith in the validity of your interpretations, and defend against anecdotalism, in that they give some perspective on how common particular kinds of views or experiences were. For instance, in this report of the problems faced by single-handed GPs, based on an interview study, Green (1993a) includes counts to indicate how common particular problems were:

> Seven single handed general practitioners mentioned problems with finding locum cover: one claimed not to have had a holiday for nine years. There were practical problems in finding reliable locums and coping financially, but some of the single handed doctors also felt unhappy about leaving 'their' practice in the hands of someone else ... five ... reported providing 24 hour cover themselves every day. ... (Green 1993a: 608)

It is not always appropriate to 'count' in this way, but some indication should be given about the typicality of, for instance, observations or particular accounts and how they have been selected from the entire data set.

Providing enough context for the reader to judge interpretations is another way of increasing credibility. Depending on the nature of the study, this could include: the interviewer's prompts, details of the research setting, the history of the research project itself, or the interactions within which the 'quote' used was observed.

Respondent validation (sometimes called *member validation*) is one method sometimes suggested as a 'validity check'. This involves taking the findings back to the participants, and ensuring that they agree. Here, the assumption is perhaps that the aim of qualitative analysis is to achieve an 'emic' understanding (see Chapter 6), and that the ultimate mark of credibility is that the researchers' and the insiders' accounts tally. There are some good reasons to feed back findings to participants: it is good manners to inform those who contributed to the study what you found; there may be issues of confidentiality you need to check; participants may want to ensure that any reports are not going to damage their interests; participants may want to make corrections in, for instance, quoted material or examples (a reliability check); and their comments on your analysis are an excellent source of further data. However, if the aims of the research are anything more than those of merely *reporting* participants' accounts of the world, respondent validation is a rather questionable exercise as a way of ensuring validity. First, the analysis might have to account for participants' views in the context of both contradictions and conflicts within a group of participants, and perhaps between them and others. More fundamentally, respondent validation presupposes a 'true' picture of the world, in which we can have more faith if two accounts (those of the researcher and the participants) coincide. Within qualitative traditions, this positivist position is rather untenable: there is no reason to suppose that participants (or a group of them) are likely to analyse their own accounts in the same ways as a researcher.

Maximizes reliability

Reliability relates to the 'repeatability' of interpretation. In qualitative work, this is often interpreted as likelihood that a similar piece of research would elicit similar kinds of themes. This kind of reliability is especially important if the research project has more than one person coding or analysing the data. However, one would not necessarily expect any two researchers to identify the same themes or codes in the data, as this to some extent depends on the analyst's interests, knowledge, theoretical approach and, ultimately, their epistemological framework. However, attention to reliability does ensure that whatever interpretation is followed through is credible, and the rationale for the codes and themes is identifiable. Ways of improving reliability include close attention to 'good practice' in fieldwork, including accurate note-taking and transcriptions, and discussing your coding with colleagues. In published papers, the credibility of your analysis is improved by including raw data, so that the reader can assess how reliable your interpretations are, and demonstrating how data are linked to interpretation.

Comparative

Comparison is what drives qualitative analysis. Comparing cases within the same data set allows us to look for regularities in the data (key themes), exceptions to these, and to build typologies. Comparing data within a case allows us to explore the contextual meaning of accounts. For instance, in a study of people's accounts of accident risks, Green (1997) found that in many interview and focus group transcripts, respondents made very different claims about what an accident was in early responses to a direct question from the ones made later in the interviews when discussing their own experiences. Early in the interviews, respondents came up with 'ideal type' definitions of accidents (such as 'an injury no one meant to happen that wasn't anyone's fault'), whereas in the context of discussing actual experiences of accidental injury they suggested definitions that utilized both intention and fault. Comparing instances across one case in the data set allowed an analysis of how such definitions were used in practice, and why.

Comparison also enables theoretical analysis to develop, as data are constantly compared with the emerging theory as they are generated. Comparing new analyses to the provisional theories and 'hunches' from preceding analyses allows the researcher to refine the emerging theory and amend it. Finally, good analysis also involves comparison of the findings with other findings from the field. This does not necessarily just include findings related to the substantive topic of interest, but from the more general social science literature that relates theoretically to the issue.

Reflexive

Reflexivity is the recognition that the researcher is part of the process of producing the data and their meanings, and a conscious reflection on that process. In positivist approaches, the researcher is ideally invisible: the aim is to remove the potential biases that an individual brings to data collection and analysis, such that the data are 'pure' and untainted by social values. In most qualitative traditions, an alternative strategy is to account explicitly for subjectivity, in exploring how the context had an impact on the research and the data arising from it. In Chapters 4 and 5 we discussed in some detail how the researcher should account for the interplay between their presence, the research context and the data produced.

In practice, the term 'reflexivity' is used in a range of ways in reports of qualitative analysis. Perhaps least useful are routine statements of the sort 'As a white, European woman I was aware of how my status had an impact on my interviews with men in a Nigerian village'. Such statements tell us nothing about how the social roles of the interviewer and the participants were constructed within the research, or how these shaped the study. At the other end of the scale are intensely personal accounts of fieldwork in which the researcher is telling their story, rather than that of the research itself. Clive Seale (1999: 160–1) cautions against this more 'confessional' style of reflexivity, in which the researcher presents themselves as somehow, through a series of blunders and self-searching, achieving a true insider status. These are, he argues, more like rhetorical claims to authenticity rather than necessarily evidence of methodological awareness. He also notes (Seale 1999: 164) the limits of reflexivity, in that we cannot of course be aware of all the subconscious ways in which our assumptions shape our approaches to research.

Between the two extremes of routine triviality and research as self-exploration are, though, some 'good practice' approaches that demonstrate a reflexive awareness of the research process and increase the rigour of analysis. Some suggestions for developing a reflexive awareness might include:

- *Methodological openness*. Being explicit about the steps taken in the data production and analysis, the decisions made, and the alternatives not pursued.
- *Theoretical openness*. The theoretical starting points and assumptions made should be addressed, and the ways in which they shaped the study accounted for.
- *Awareness of the social setting of the research itself*. In interviews, or participatory fieldwork, the 'data' are largely the results of interactions between the researcher and the researched. Reflexivity requires a constant awareness of this, and the ways in which the data result from these particular interactions.
- *Awareness of the wider social context*. This might include awareness of how political and social values have both made possible the research (in whose interests is it funded?) and constrained it, and how the historical and policy contexts shape the data.

These are, at one level, a courtesy to the reader, who can then judge the findings presented in terms of the context for themselves. Beyond that, though, these are essential to thorough analysis, in that they are ways of taking seriously the elements of a qualitative approach outlined in Chapter 1.

Rigour is not enough . . .

Addressing these elements of transparency, validity, reliability, comparison and reflexivity will help produce credible analysis that is less likely to leave a sceptical reader asking 'How do I know this is not just your subjective interpretation?' However, to return to the initial discussion about imagination as well as technical skills, rigour is not enough. To begin with, the data have to support detailed analysis. However thorough and rigorous the analysis, if the data consist of nothing more than notes of brief interviews, or comments on a questionnaire, it will be difficult to generate much of explanatory power. From her perspective as a journal editor, Janice Morse (2002) complains of the dangers of 'thin' data, such as those derived from semi-structured interviews or notes written under the 'any other comments?' section of a questionnaire, which are then categorized as 'themes' and reported with no links to theory. The resulting analysis, Morse suggests, is inevitably 'shallow and trivial', with none of the rich descriptive narrative that would characterize good qualitative analysis (Morse 2002). So, a precondition of good analysis is, inevitably, good data.

Second, however thorough the analysis, if it remains at the level of superficially attaching 'codes' derived from interviewees' own accounts, with little attempt to integrate these into existing theory, or to look for connections within the data, the result will look 'under-analysed' and rather trivial. This may suffice if working in a new field, or with participants whose voices are rarely heard, in which case simply reporting views is the aim in itself. However, this does not quite count as 'qualitative analysis'. The key to producing insightful, satisfying accounts of 'what is going on' in your data is to bring a social science imagination to it: to identify connections both within the data and between them and the world outside. This is far harder to achieve than simply analysing in a rigorous and systematic way, and it is perhaps impossible to be prescriptive about how to achieve satisfying as well as rigorous analysis. However, there are ways of increasing the depth of your data analysis, and some suggestions for developing an imaginative approach are:

- Read and discuss widely – not just within your own topic and discipline, but from other disciplines, to look for connections and transferable concepts.
- Ask constantly about the context of the data: think about them in terms of historical, political, social and cultural contexts.
- Return frequently to the theoretical assumptions embedded in your research question (see Chapter 2): challenge them, think about how different assumptions might provide a fresh look at what is going on.
- Interrogate your data with colleagues: other people will have a different reading of your data, and may challenge your common-sense accounts of what is going on. Equally, helping others with their data analysis can help encourage a more imaginative approach to your own.

Generalizability and transferability

A final issue in qualitative analysis is that of generalizability. Generalizability refers to the extent to which findings from a study apply to a wider population or to different contexts. In a sample survey, random sampling allows generalizability through the principle that the study sample is likely to be statistically representative of the larger population of interest, so findings can be extrapolated to that population. In qualitative work, study participants are rarely randomly sampled in this way, and the logic of generalizability is rather different. Some argue that it is not an issue in qualitative work, which properly aims to provide 'thick' description, or to address particularities, rather than to provide 'typical' accounts or generalizable findings.

There are, though, two reasons why researchers in the field of health do have to address the issue of generalizability. First, if researchers are to make claims to their findings being useful, at whatever level, to health practice, they do have to consider the theoretical import of their findings: the extent to which they refer to some setting or population wider than that of the research itself. Second, and more pragmatically, the credibility of qualitative findings in non-social science fields is often fragile, and qualitative research is easily marginalized as 'interesting, but not research evidence' because the generalizability is questionable. Addressing these concerns does not mean adopting, or even adapting, the procedures of quantitative approaches and attempting to imitate the kinds of random samples drawn, or comparing the study population to wider ones. Instead, it involves thinking through what *kind of relationship* the study findings have to other populations and settings, and unpacking exactly what inferences can be drawn from the data analysis.

Essentially, though, these all refer to the same question that generalizability addresses in quantitative work; namely, how far can the findings of this particular study be extrapolated? There are various ways in which findings from qualitative work can be supported as more widely relevant. These include:

Sensitizing concepts

If researching relatively under-researched topics, or respondents, the issue of generalizability may be less salient than that of 'sensitizing' readers to new ways of thinking, or the potential views of respondents. In Case Study 1.1, for instance, the researchers found that many of the 'asthma' patients they interviewed did not believe they had asthma. At one level, it doesn't matter how representative their sample was of the whole population: the key point is that practitioners are sensitized to the fact that *some* patients may not accept the diagnosis. At a more theoretical level, qualitative studies may generate concepts that are 'good to think with', and thus have a utility beyond their immediate research setting in sensitizing other researchers to useful concepts. Case Study 1.1 made use of the concept of 'stigma', from Erving Goffman's work on the impact of stigmatizing attributes on social interaction (Goffman 1963). In Goffman's original study, it perhaps matters little how far his data are representative of the population, or whether the findings can be generalized in an empirical sense: what matters is the theoretical usefulness of the concepts (such as stigma) he developed, which have been used widely in qualitative research. This suggests that the most appropriate way of thinking about generalizability in qualitative work is in terms of *conceptual generalizability*.

Conceptual generalizability

The key elements that are generalizable from qualitative analysis may not be the narrow findings, but the concepts; that is, the ways of thinking about or 'making sense' of the world. These concepts, whether at macro or 'middle' level (see Chapter 2), might inform understanding of similar contexts or issues. Goffman's work on stigma is an obvious example from the 'classic' literature in medical sociology, but this also applies to more recent and more applied work. For example, in Chapter 1, one of the examples of qualitative research studies cited in Box 1.1 was Joseph Opala and François Boillot's ethnographic study of traditional beliefs about leprosy among the Limba. Here, the question of generalizability is not 'How far are the beliefs they identified typical of other groups, or the whole population of Sierra Leone?' but rather 'How far do these findings help us understand what is going on when in situations where biomedicine meets traditional beliefs?' As Opala and Boillot (1996) note, workers in the field of leprosy are interested in studies of traditional beliefs, as they recognize that effective health care can only be provided when the user's perspective is taken into account. The 'generalizable' findings of Opala and Boillot are that to do this adequately relies on a detailed understanding of not just beliefs about leprosy, but also an understanding of the world-view of which these beliefs form a part. In their study, which explored why different groups of Limba had different attitudes to the stigma of leprosy, they found that there were considerable variations in terms of views of traditional and biomedical treatments and when to take medicines. The specifics of beliefs about medications are not generalizable, but the *concept* that there are local variations, and these are important for health care workers to identify, is. Similarly, they found a number of misconceptions that medical workers held about local beliefs. These included the idea that local people believed leprosy was caused by eating one's totem, or that the majority used traditional medicines. Neither of these beliefs was supported by the research evidence, and to 'counter' non-existent beliefs in health promotion messages might well be counter-productive. Again, these specific misconceptions may not be generalizable, but the general point (that we should focus on medical workers' ideas of lay health beliefs, as well as the health beliefs themselves) is.

Transferability

Here, the question is 'To what extent are these findings transferable to other settings?' This is what the practitioner or policy-maker reading your report is going to want to know: is this something I can apply to my clinic, or my patients, or my country? Answering this question relies on thinking through what is context specific, and what might be more widely applicable within the findings. To return to Opala and Boillot's (1996) study, they also discuss the transferability of their recommendations. Opala and Boillot are able to draw out a transferable strategy for shaping health promotion messages, involving identifying medical workers' misconceptions about local beliefs, focusing on the differences between local and medical beliefs, and using indigenous knowledge to provide analogies to use in health promotion.

Conclusion

Qualitative researchers working in the field of health have to pay rather more attention to the mechanics of data analysis than has perhaps been traditional in mainstream social science disciplines. This has had some benefits, not least in generating discussion around how we demonstrate the credibility of our interpretations, and ensure that analysis is done rigorously and thoroughly. However, we have also suggested that the application of practical techniques is not sufficient for producing insightful and useful qualitative findings. Researchers also have to ground their analyses in a broad-ranging understanding of theoretical and other empirical work in their discipline in order to bring a 'social science' imagination to their own data.

KEY POINTS

- To provide credible findings for health, qualitative researchers need to address questions of reliability, validity and generalizability.
- There are a number of approaches to analysis, and in practice most researchers use a pragmatic mix of techniques.
- Whatever style of analysis is adopted, it is important to be explicit about the methods used and rigorous in their application.
- Moving beyond merely descriptive accounts of data entails an imaginative as well as a rigorous approach to data analysis.

EXERCISES

1 Take an example of published qualitative work, and consider whether you found the report credible and interesting. Then identify what techniques the authors have used in their analysis that contributed to your answer: did they provide context, were they transparent about the methods used, were they reflexive?

2   The only way to develop skills in analysis is to practise doing it. This exercise requires a short extract from an interview transcript. If you don't have any data of your own, ask colleagues for an extract (suitably anonymized) to use. Take two or three pages, and first identify any 'themes' that you feel might be emerging. Code the text by 'marking it up' in the margins, with each theme labelled as a code.

Next, try 'open coding' the extract, using the techniques of grounded theory introduced in this chapter. Ask a series of questions about each line of the data: What is going on here? How can we label that as a provisional concept? Are there in vivo codes? What are the properties and dimensions of the concepts that are emerging? Draw on your experience and reading to provide comparisons for each provisional concept, to aid this process. If possible, do this exercise in a group with colleagues. Compare your original list of themes with the provisional list of concepts generated by the open coding exercise.

FURTHER READING

Strauss, A. (1987) *Qualitative analysis for social scientists*. Cambridge: Cambridge University Press. Detailed account of principles of grounded theory, quoting extensively from Glaser and Strauss's book *The discovery of grounded theory* (1967). This has extended examples taken from student and research team seminars on coding and analysis, taking the reader through common problems faced by researchers. Essential reading for anyone planning on developing skills in the grounded theory approach.

Seale, C. (1999) *The quality of qualitative research*. London: Sage. Clive Seale discusses various methodological positions on issues such as validity, reliability and generalizability and provides some practical approaches to maximizing the quality and credibility of qualitative analysis.

Miles, M.B. and Huberman, A.M. (1994) *Qualitative data analysis: an expanded sourcebook* (2nd ed.). Thousand Oaks, CA: Sage. Full of practical suggestions for organizing, analysing and presenting qualitative data. Miles and Huberman have a pragmatic approach that uses a range of methods for coding, comparing cases and thinking about the relationships in your data. Many of these are graphic, using data matrices to sort and display data.

Part 3

Doing Qualitative Work for Health

9

Collaborating Across Disciplines and Institutions

CHAPTER SUMMARY

Few health researchers work in isolation, and qualitative health research is often conducted in the context of multi-disciplinary programmes, and research collaborations also require us to work across national boundaries and institutional settings. These kinds of collaborations bring both challenges and opportunities. There are various models of how researchers from different disciplinary backgrounds can and should work together.

Introduction

Academic research in all disciplines is increasingly likely to be a collaborative venture (Godin and Gingras 2000). Rather than working as a lone researcher, with sole responsibility for research design, data collection, analysis and dissemination, qualitative researchers contributing to health research programmes typically work as members of collaborative teams. These teams may be based in multi-disciplinary departments, and many projects span a number of collaborating institutions and perhaps countries. Researchers do not just collaborate with academics from other disciplines, but may also be developing partnerships with non-academics such as non-governmental organizations or health service providers. There are, in many countries, policies in place that actively promote various kinds of collaborative working, for instance those that encourage academic researchers to work with those in industrial and non-governmental sectors, and to work with end-point users of the research findings, such as service providers and clients. There are certainly a number of incentives for researchers to work collaboratively. In a world of increasing information, and access to information, it is very difficult for the individual researcher to keep abreast even of developments in their own field, let alone those in related fields. Collaboration, in theory, increases the 'efficiency' of research effort, through building information and dissemination networks. Working with users and those placed to implement findings can also increase the 'effectiveness' of research, particularly for those working in policy- and practice-relevant areas. Planning research in collaboration with end-point users, rather than merely disseminating results to them at the end of a project, is perhaps more likely to ensure that research resonates with users' needs. There are also potential gains in terms of capacity-building, in that international collaborations can help spread the skills and infrastructure needed to develop local research capacity, and collaborations with health professionals can raise awareness of and skills in qualitative methodologies.

However, collaboration of any kind brings a number of challenges. Most researchers have learned their craft within a particular discipline, in a particular country, in which both formal and informal norms about research practice are acquired. Fundamental ideas about what research is for, and how we can produce valid knowledge, are closely tied to the kinds of epistemological orientations we introduced in Chapter 1, and those of qualitative research may not be shared by those trained in other traditions. The ways in which qualitative researchers address questions of research design, such as how to identify a credible sample, or what methods are appropriate for producing the data, may be unfamiliar to those more comfortable with more quantitative, positivist paradigms. The norms of 'good ethical practice', despite international guidelines, are to some extent locally specific, as we discussed in Chapter 3. Even expectations around how research protocols should be written are culturally shaped. There is some evidence, for instance, that deductive styles (in which the main point is introduced first, followed by information that supports it, or provides context) are preferred in Britain, whereas Asian writers feel more comfortable with inductive styles that lead up to the main point late in the protocol (Cortazzi and Jin 1997: 81). Differences in research practice, epistemology or style are of course rarely neutral, and qualitative researchers often face the challenge of having to 'defend' their approaches in institutions or programmes in which more positivist paradigms are the norm. Good working relationships across national, institutional or disciplinary boundaries cannot be assumed just because individual members of the team are committed to joint working. The experience of most researchers is that partnerships need considerable time and effort to develop.

Different methods for different questions

In Chapter 2, we outlined some of the ways in which qualitative studies are used in conjunction with other research designs to build our understanding of health issues. In practice, much applied health research requires a number of different approaches to data collection within one study, especially if the study is supporting a public health intervention of some kind. If you look back at Case Study 1.2, for instance, quantitative methods were needed to address the *effectiveness* of the Kopana intervention (did it increase the number of TB treatments completed?) whereas qualitative methods were needed to explore *why* the intervention did or did not work. The problems facing public health are increasingly complex, and require a range of methodological strategies to research adequately (Baum 1995). Identifying needs for interventions might typically require qualitative work alongside epidemiological surveys to assess need, and then a mixed method approach to evaluating the intervention, in for instance using epidemiological methods to measure outcomes (such as disease incidence) and qualitative methods to explore process and users' views of the intervention. The example in Case Study 9.1 illustrates this mixed methods approach in the context of one public health issue, that of increasing the uptake of insecticide-treated bed nets.

This example of how a variety of qualitative and quantitative methods were used in one programme is perhaps typical of public health interventions that require both a range of data to support implementation, and a flexibility of approaches to respond to the early stages of evaluation. The participatory evaluation of the Stepping Stones sexual health programme in The Gambia, described in Case Study 2.2, is another example of this kind of flexible evaluation in a public health setting. These examples illustrate perhaps the simplest model of interdisciplinary working, in which different methods are used to address specific research questions raised by the study, and the skills of a multi-disciplinary team are brought in as 'experts' in the particular methodological approaches needed. Ideally, findings from each component of the programme inform each other as it progresses.

Multiple methods: to increase understanding or increase validity?

Using multiple methods within the same project is, then, common-sense good practice if the study addresses a number of distinct research questions, for which different methodological approaches are implicated. In this case, the qualitative component may be to all practical purposes a 'stand-alone' project, with its own management and methods, and the process separate from other projects within the study. However, most multi-disciplinary projects aim to gain 'added value' from including a number of components, in the hope that the findings from each will feed into a broader understanding

Case Study 9.1   Multi-disciplinary approaches in an intervention to promote insecticide-treated bed nets

(Source: Winch, P. (1999) 'The role of anthropological methods in a community-based mosquito net intervention in Bagamoyo District, Tanzania', in R. Hahn (ed.), *Anthropology in public health: bridging differences in culture and society*. Oxford: Oxford University Press, pp. 44–62)

Peter Winch (1999) discusses the wide range of research questions that the promotion of insecticide-treated bed nets instigates. These bed nets, used regularly, are seen as a vital element in reducing the transmission of malaria in endemic areas. Based on one community-based intervention in Bagamoyo District, Tanzania, Winch describes a series of studies that were all designed to address questions about how bed net use could be encouraged. In Bagamoyo District malaria is endemic and predominantly affects young children and pregnant women, with about half of all deaths under four years old being due to malaria, and iron-deficiency anaemia (one result of malaria infection) affecting most children. The Bagamoyo Bed Net Project used a multi-method approach to address three related research questions:

Why did villagers not view malaria control as a high priority?
How could year-round bed net use be encouraged?
How could retreatment of nets with insecticide be encouraged?

To access local views of malaria, researchers used the methods of ethnographic interviewing. At community meetings, to which local teachers, health workers and others were invited, the researchers used two techniques to elicit local terms for illness – free listing and pile sorting. Free listing involves asking participants to list all types of a phenomenon (such as illnesses, risks to health, or symptoms of malaria), prompting for more until an exhaustive list is produced. Pile sorting requires these items to be listed on cards, asking participants to sort the cards into piles of similar terms, and to justify how they have grouped them. These introductory meetings were followed up with interviews (individual and group) in which respondents were asked to provide descriptions of each illness, along with symptoms and how it is treated. Finally, all the terms that were compatible with malaria were used in a sample survey of all villagers. Local classifications of illnesses did not map onto biomedical classifications, with only some of the illness defined as 'malaria' in biomedical terms seen as dangerous. One local illness term, *degedege*, classified as malaria by the researchers but not the local people, described a feared disease of sudden onset, severe fever and high mortality. This was described as being caused by a spirit that attacked children. This was only identified as caused by malaria when it occurred during the rainy season, when mosquitoes are numerous. This finding suggested one reason why villagers may not use the bed nets throughout the year, as intended: if malaria is only seen as a disease of the rainy season, there are few incentives to use them at other times of the year. The anthropological research also revealed that some of the illnesses that would be seen as malaria by medical workers were seen as relatively unimportant by local people. This fed into interventions designed to alert villagers to the consequences of malaria, such as tiredness and poor outcomes in pregnancy. Health promotion messages were promoted through plays that informed villagers about the effects of malaria, and calendars to remind them of the importance of using nets the whole year round.

After these interventions, the research team carried out a household survey of a systematic sample of households to count the number of bed nets owned by the household and how often they were used by household members. One aim of the survey was to evaluate the health promotion messages developed from the anthropological research. The researchers counted how many nets were used in each household, and identified a number of problems: that there was still a perception that malaria was not a problem during the dry season, and that women and older children often had no access to bed nets. Talking to householders also identified some practical barriers, such as the problem of men travelling to the city during the dry season for work, and taking bed nets with them.

Finally, interviews and participant observation were used in a third study to look at barriers to the retreatment of bed nets with insecticide. Interviews revealed some of the barriers: cost, inconvenience, and worries about the toxicity of the insecticide. Participant observation in the villages provided an important context for understanding which householders were getting their nets retreated, in that some groups in the villages had strong leadership and a high level of social cohesion, with both strong support for the retreatment programme and the network of relationships that enabled retreatment to be paid for.

Winch comments that the key advantages of anthropological methods were their flexibility, in a project that had a number of aims and research questions. A mix of methods allowed different questions raised by the intervention and its evaluation to be addressed as they were needed.

of the topic studied, or increase the validity of the findings from all contributing studies.

Following on from the discussion of epistemological approaches in Chapter 1, there are two models of how this can happen. The first assumes that there are a range of (theoretically informed) questions raised by the consideration of any health problem, and that different research designs will be needed to address them. Here, the different methodological approaches are seen as 'adding depth', such that the whole research programme moves towards a richer understanding. If using multiple methods for adding depth is relatively straightforward (at least in principle – we come to some problems below), a second model for using multiple methods within one study is perhaps rather more contentious. This is the idea of *triangulation*, or using more than one method to increase our faith in the validity of findings.

The notion of triangulation borrows a metaphor from navigation, with the idea that taking two readings will enable us to pinpoint the 'truth' more accurately than one. Thus, one method of data collection can be used to offset the weakness of another, or to 'check out' the validity of findings. Examples might include the use of other data sources to 'validate' behavioural accounts from interview data: using sales figures for contraceptives, for instance, to compare with interview reports of contraceptive use, or medical records to check interviewees' accounts of medication prescriptions. However, there are of course limits to how far we can use different strategies for collecting data to improve the 'accuracy' of those data. Clearly, looking at sales of contraceptives and asking people about the use of contraceptives are generating data about two rather different phenomena. Less contentious is the use of triangulation to provide another perspective on a particular phenomenon, or 'fill in the gaps', for instance by using oral history interviews to complement historical documentary research. Norman Denzin (1989b) discusses the possibilities of triangulation from a more qualitative perspective; that is, that validity might refer to an improved understanding, rather than improved 'accuracy'. He argues that triangulation does not necessarily imply a naïve positivist position, in which one can more accurately pin down some reality that is the object of research, but rather an approach that can bring the object more sharply into focus:

> ... each method implies a different line of action toward reality – and hence each will reveal different aspects of it, much as a kaleidoscope, depending on the angle at which it is held, will reveal different colours and configurations of objects to the viewer. Methods are like the kaleidoscope: depending on how they are approached, held, and acted toward, different observations will be revealed. (Denzin 1989b: 235)

Thus, the aim is not to produce a consistent version of the object of study, as that object is always socially constructed, but to offset the particular weaknesses of each method, and challenge the biases that come from only one perspective. As an example, look again at Case Study 2.1, which described how Hilary Graham used both interviews and diaries in her study of women and smoking. Note that the diaries were not used to 'validate' women's interview accounts of the number of cigarettes smoked, but were used to generate slightly different information, and that these differences were what helped Graham unpack the meanings of smoking for the women in her study.

For Denzin, triangulation of methods is only one possible strategy. We can also use data triangulation (in utilizing as many diverse sources of data as possible), investigator triangulation (using different observers) and, most challenging, the idea of theoretical triangulation. This involves widening the theoretical frameworks utilized in a study as the research progresses, such that a range of models and theories are at the forefront when analysing the empirical data collected. It is with Denzin's idea of theoretical triangulation that researchers in multi-disciplinary health studies are perhaps at a particular advantage. Most public health projects can draw on the theoretical traditions of a number of disciplines, widening the potential interpretative frameworks to be used in analysis. However, in practice, few health projects utilize the possibilities of theoretical triangulation.

In considering the implications of 'mixing methods' in health promotion research, for instance, Kathryn Milburn and colleagues (Milburn et al. 1995) argue that in much health promotion research, methods are combined uncritically, with little consideration of exactly what was to be achieved by using them together. This applies, perhaps, to health research more generally. Combining methods is assumed to be 'a good thing', an end in itself, and there is often insufficient attention paid to the relationships between the various components:

> ... are the researchers concerned about ... choosing methods for their appropriateness to the topic and the purpose of the research? Or are they concerned with 'illumination', and therefore with using different methods sequentially, the one to inform the other? Alternatively, are they concerned with 'saturation', with several methods being used simultaneously either to verify or augment the findings of each single approach? Or is there concern with 'diversification', so that several approaches are used in order to tap multiple realities in a particular setting? (Milburn et al. 1995: 348)

They advise clarity on exactly what is to be achieved in using a number of methodological approaches within one project. Given the varying expectations those from different disciplinary backgrounds can have about the relative contributions of different methodological strategies, the partners in any collaboration may well have to spend considerable time in exploring these differences to reduce the risk of frustration when outputs do not 'fit together' in the predicted way.

Trans-disciplinary work

One approach to multi-disciplinary work is, then, to be explicit about the epistemological differences within the team, and to highlight the range of expectations about the separate contributions of each of the partners. Another is to try to move towards a shared approach – a more 'trans-disciplinary' model. Here, the aim is to integrate the different theoretical and methodological insights from each discipline throughout the project, rather than at the point of combining the findings. For some researchers, the division of labour between epidemiologists, anthropologists and clinicians is an artificial and unhelpful one that should be struggled against: they are, in this light, 'natural partners'.

Yach (1992), for instance, points out that health research has traditionally used mixed methods and integrated research designs in public health settings, and only with the rise of laboratory studies in the late nineteenth century did the social researchers decline in importance. The separation of specialities in health research is, then, relatively recent and there has been a long history of integrated work. He cites as an example the Polela Health Unit in South Africa, which from 1940 was based on primary health care principles using both social science and epidemiological methods to assess the local population's health status. Yach argues that the walls that have been built up between the disciplines, in which each has its own journals, conferences and particular language, are unhelpful and he urges greater integration in public health training.

This call for a more integrative approach is echoed by Marcia Inhorn (1995), who notes that few health research projects really achieve collaborative efforts, in part because anthropologists have some rather fixed ideas about the gulf between epidemiology and anthropology: that, for instance, epidemiologists are reductionist, tied to biomedical ideas about disease and not sensitive to social complexity. Many of the assumptions, she says, are misguided, and the apparent gaps between the two disciplines are a reason to develop collaborations, rather than resist them. In this model of trans–disciplinary working, differences between disciplines are seen as productive. Through challenging our assumptions about both our own disciplines and those of other partners in the collaboration, we can identify how each can contribute in a more integrated approach.

This vision of a coming together of social and health sciences is an appealing one, and 'breaking down barriers' is difficult to argue against without appearing elitist or protectionist about one's own discipline. However, it does perhaps ignore the 'political economy' of public health research, in which the research agenda tends to be set by those from particular health professions, and not social scientists, and is perhaps naïve about the epistemological (rather than merely methodological) differences between the contributing disciplines. Often, pleas for 'breaking down the barriers' appear to be little more than exasperated requests for anthropologists or sociologists to do the fieldwork that public health specialists want doing, rather than genuine collaborations around research agenda, and research questions (see Pelto and Pelto's 1992 complaint about the paucity of trained social scientists for applied health research in developing countries for one example of this). As we have seen, the theoretical and epistemological starting points for research will shape the kinds of questions seen as legitimate, and what methods will produce valid answers to those research questions. In this light, anthropologists may well be reluctant to contribute to yet another 'rapid appraisal', considering the data collected is a poor guide to local beliefs (see Chapter 6).

There are of course many examples of such collaborations working well, and Case Study 6.1, on using ethnography in a diarrhoeal disease project, demonstrates the possibilities of informing public interventions on the basis of ethnographic work. But productive multi–disciplinary work does not just happen: it requires considerable planning. In their reports of the project described in Case Study 6.1, the authors discuss some of the reasons for anthropological perspectives being successfully integrated into practice (Scrimshaw and Hurtado 1988), including building on a field prepared by earlier anthropologists who had worked in Central America, the receptivity of project staff, and care taken to prepare reports and findings in useful formats for non-specialists, especially using face-to-face meetings to explore how they could be used in the project. As Scrimshaw and Hurtado (1988) note, this is time-consuming and resource-intensive. In many studies, researchers are too busy with the next project to consider appropriate dissemination formats, or to explore the implications of their findings for practice. Susan Rifkin (1996) also notes that there are unexpectedly time-consuming parts of the 'rapid' appraisal process, and she suggests it can take a long time to develop the research objectives if the team do not share a common language or approach, and a new shared one has to be developed. Rifkin (1996) suggests that visualizations are one way in which members of teams can share ideas more easily: using diagrams and rankings to get across key points in ways that are not tied to disciplinary ways of thinking. In the diarrhoeal disease project, Scrimshaw and Hurtado used typologies of ethnoclassifications to introduce other members of the team to the basic concepts, rather than extensive written reports.

Communicating across disciplines

It is not only in rapid appraisals that problems of communication can be a barrier to productive working across disciplines. In Case Study 9.2, Gillian Lewando-Hundt (2000) describes the different expectations of various stakeholders in a project on maternal and child health around such issues as how to disseminate findings in appropriate ways.

In this case, political sensitivities as well as disciplinary traditions created challenges. The political sensitivities of working in the Middle East mean that such difficulties were particularly acute in this project, but similar challenges face most multi-disciplinary projects in the dissemination phase. Some typical areas of tension faced within many research teams include:

- *Publications.* Researchers from particular disciplines will be keen to publish in 'their' journals. Although most large projects furnish enough findings for several publications, it is helpful to have discussions at the outset of the project about who will take the lead on which publications, who will contribute to particular papers (and have authorship) and where the project findings will be disseminated. (Authorship is discussed further in Chapter 10.)
- *Ownership of the data.* On a large, collaborative project, writing up will probably continue long after the project itself has finished. Again, it is essential to be clear at the outset who will have access to whatever data have been generated at the end of the project, and who will have 'rights' to exploit those data.
- *Outputs.* Given the flexibility of qualitative designs, the research 'answers' that come out may not be the ones expected. It is not uncommon for a key finding of qualitative studies to be that the original research question was the 'wrong' question. In a stand-alone project, this is not a problem, but in collaborative projects, with research partners perhaps reliant on the qualitative phase to

Case Study 9.2   Collaborations across disciplines and nations: problems of language and politics

(Source: Lewando-Hundt, G. (2000) 'Multiple scripts and contested discourse in disseminating research findings', *Social Policy and Administration*, 34: 419–33)

Gillian Lewando-Hundt reports on some of the challenges in disseminating research findings from a study of maternal and child health to Palestinians in Gaza and Bedouin in Israel. The study was funded by the European Commission as a collaboration between universities in the UK and Israel and a research centre in Palestine, and included researchers trained in epidemiology and public health, some of whom also had service responsibilities, and anthropologists. Lewando-Hundt argues that the different national, disciplinary and research orientations of the team led to different understandings throughout the project of issues around study design, interpretation of the results and dissemination. These can be a productive force for developing research questions. In this study, the members of the team with responsibility for service provision and a public health perspective wanted to focus on non-attenders at pre-natal clinics, and find out whether they were informed about the service on offer and why they did not attend. From a more social science perspective, the anthropologists were more comfortable asking questions about professional and client views and experiences, and focusing on what the women gained or did not gain by attending. These differences in focus were accommodated by dividing the research questions according to methodology, such that the epidemiologists led on designing a questionnaire survey to measure service utilization, and the anthropologists developed qualitative studies using focus groups and interviews to explore users' views and experiences (one of these studies is described in Case Study 5.1). By conducting both quantitative and qualitative studies as part of the same project, the two disciplines could see that using a combination of methods provided answers to slightly different questions, but both contributed to understanding the issue of maternal and child health.

When it came to dissemination, there were also differences across the research team in terms of expectations about what was legitimate. As an EC-funded study, the co-ordinators had an obligation to disseminate widely, but this did not form part of the normal expectations of the local research teams in Gaza and Israel, where the accepted process was to move on to planning interventions, without a lengthy phase of dissemination. The challenges of disseminating the key findings included difficulties of addressing diverse audiences, and conflict over which languages to write it in. The Palestinians were keen to have Arabic translations to disseminate widely in an accessible format, whereas one member of the team wanted a more limited dissemination, and only in English. In the end the draft report was summarized and translated into both Arabic and Hebrew, with these as well as the English versions bound into one document.

Expectations around the format of dissemination also led to conflicts. When the researchers first presented some of the qualitative data from the focus groups, they included data on women's views of the issue of *wasta*, or using influence or connections to jump the queue. They had intended this to be a way of informing health centre managers and others about the key findings, and generating discussion about the implications. However, the sensitivities about the topic (*wasta*) and the lack of understanding of the methods (group interviews) meant that the findings were challenged by the audience, who commented that the methods were unscientific, and the data could not be believed. In another meeting, the researchers were advised to tone down some of the criticisms reported of the clinics, and to use the word 'social' rather than 'political'. Some of the particular difficulties faced were the result of political tensions in the Middle East, but Lewando-Hundt suggests that all dissemination strategies have to take account of the ethos of local health services, the sensitivities of the various groups involved, and their expectations about what data 'should' look like.

Political sensitivities also shaped how findings were disseminated in academic journals. For instance, although the context for the Gaza setting was health service provision by the Israeli Civil Administration, this was usually too contentious to note. Direct comment by the authors on the position of Palestinians was avoided, in case it appeared to be politically biased, and they instead quoted other authors. Choosing whether to use Hebrew or Arabic names for places, or whether to use the term 'Bedouin', 'Bedouin Arabs', 'Palestinian Israelis' or 'Israeli Arabs', was not just a matter of linguistic preference, but one that suggested particular political affiliations. For joint papers, a compromise had to be reached on terminology, with drafts being discussed by members of the research team until consensus was reached.

In this study, then, not only disciplinary differences but also political and institutional differences had to be negotiated throughout the research process. Although these issues might be particularly explicit in settings in transition, such as the Middle East, they are likely to shape research in most collaborative settings, and we have to pay attention not just to the technical aspects of research design, but also to the politics of research.

---

provide data for their contribution, colleagues can find this extremely frustrating. Writing up these unexpected findings (and explaining why the aims may not have been met in expected ways) can present dilemmas for the project team.

- *Language.* Even if teams are working in the same language, disciplines still have their own vocabularies, with terms that have specific meanings. 'Observational study' means something rather different to epidemiologists and sociologists, for instance. Further, the concepts used in health research may carry quite different connotations across different disciplines. Clinicians, for instance, may be comfortable with the concept of 'lay perceptions' to distinguish their patients' understanding of health from their professional, biomedical ideas. However, for many sociologists and anthropologists the term implies that lay and expert beliefs are distinct and that lay ones are somehow 'faulty', so terms such as 'public views' may be preferred. In collaborative projects, if all partners are expected to agree to the wording of all outputs, the time taken to reach consensus around terminology can be considerable.

If we assume that the contribution of qualitative research is to bring methodological expertise to address particular research questions, these practical differences between disciplinary research cultures can be addressed, given adequate time for teamwork and debate. However, there are perhaps more fundamental differences in the epistemological starting points of many of the social sciences and the more biomedical sciences, which can potentially be more undermining of fruitful collaboration. Within health research programmes addressing a 'public health problem', the agenda is perhaps inevitably set in biomedical terms, and if bringing a social science approach, rather than just qualitative methods, many qualitative researchers will feel rather uncomfortable with an uncritical biomedical perspective. Robert Pool (1994), for instance, reflects on the tensions raised by the 'biomedical' framework he had to adopt in order to fund anthropological research on health and illness in Cameroon:

> The goal of my original research project was to discover the cultural factors related to infant nutrition and illness. ... These insights were to lead to recommendations for improving infant nutrition. ... [However] I was opposed to the idea that the anthropologist studying health related beliefs should adopt an evaluative attitude based on biomedical assumptions. Rather, I preferred to explore people's ideas about illness and food and place them in a wider cultural context. However, grant-giving agencies desired a more applied approach. ... (Pool 1994: 27–9)

Pool was working in an area where local health workers considered kwashiorkor (protein-energy malnutrition) to be a major health problem. From a biomedical perspective, the 'causes' of this problem were perceived to be dysfunctional health beliefs and practices, which could be identified through anthropological methods. However, as Pool notes, this sits rather uneasily within a broader anthropological perspective, which would aim for holistic understanding of local culture without a priori assumptions about the validity of local health workers' ideas about causation.

In her critique of the 'natural collaboration' model for anthropology and epidemiology, Susan DiGiacomo (1999) is rather pessimistic about the possibilities of genuinely collaborative partnerships between the disciplines. She outlines a number of assumptions made by epidemiological science that lead her to question whether there could ever be a 'cultural epidemiology'. First, she argues, epidemiology, with its 'web of causation' model, tends to reify culture as simply one more risk factor to be accounted for in models of epidemiological risk. Disease incidence is merely the sum of individual cases of disease, and culture reduced to a list of 'social' factors (age, sex, race) that are similarly individualized as attributes of particular people in particular places. A more holistic, anthropological notion of culture is difficult to maintain against this reductionist concept. She identifies five underlying assumptions in epidemiology which are at odds with anthropological practice:

1 It is possible to isolate cultural concepts from their context.
2 Culture can be reified as 'value', 'attitudes' and 'beliefs' and these can be attached to particular social groups.
3 Culture is a 'risk factor', even if a protective one.
4 Culture is an attribute of 'others', defined in terms of ethnicity, or social class.
5 The beliefs of these 'others' tend to be unreasonable, irrational and in need of explanation.

DiGiacomo argues that the stress on methods, rather than theory, in the intersection of anthropology and epidemiology has reduced anthropologists to merely data-gatherers, with the focus on collecting information on these cultural 'beliefs' rather than producing 'thick descriptions' that provide the context and holistic understanding needed to interpret the meaning of beliefs. She also notes that it is not just epistemological differences that constrain the role of anthropology within epidemiology, but also institutional pressures. Spain, where she was based, like many other countries, puts pressure on its academic departments to publish in high-impact journals in a narrow range, and not more imaginative pieces in social science journals. As she concludes:

> The requirements ... of genuinely collaborative work go well beyond matters of epistemology to include the politics of scientific research, and demand some degree of courage from all concerned, but especially from epidemiologists in pursuing lines of research that do not necessarily promise fast returns with high bibliographic impact value. (DiGiacomo 1999: 451)

Projects involving partners from a number of disciplinary backgrounds involve, then, at a minimum, challenges in terms of working across varying communication and research cultures. They can also raise more fundamental challenges of addressing epistemological differences, and developing research agendas that accommodate social science as well as biomedical or epidemiological perspectives.

International collaborations

International projects range from studies based in one country that use data from another, through to major international collaborations with research management spanning several continents. Jessica Ogden and John Porter

(2000) point to the rhetoric of collaboration for international public health, and criticize a simplistic notion of 'partnership' to describe international collaborations, given the inequalities of power between research institutes in the north and south. In their examples, from collaborations between institutions in the UK and India, they argue that it is important to separate out relationships between institutions and those between individual researchers or research teams, and distinguish both from short-term 'consultancy' relationships, in which researchers spend time in other countries as technical experts, working to the agenda of the host institution. Institutions may have a formal collaborative agreement, but this only becomes a partnership in practice if individuals within the research team can develop a collaborative working relationship. Individual power differences between members of the research teams, in terms of seniority or the relative status of their discipline, can undermine collaborative working. Ogden and Porter also point to structural barriers to collaboration. The costs of research can vary considerably between countries, with those in the UK five to ten times higher than those of the Indian institutions. This creates an image of the northern partners being 'worth more', which is hardly conducive to partnership.

Cultures of communication vary across national boundaries, as well as across disciplines. Martin Cortazzi and Lixian Jin (1997) discuss the impact of different communication cultures on teaching and learning for students, but many of their points apply equally well to research collaborations. First, there are different academic cultures that frame our expectations of what 'good' research and academic activity look like. Experienced research practitioners come to think of these as obvious and universal, but they do vary from country to country. Thus, our expectations of whether team relationships should be hierarchical, 'master–disciple' or collegial, or whether persuasive rhetoric is an essential element of professional skills, will depend on our cultural background. How far junior members of a team are expected to show originality, creativity or critical skills also varies across cultures, as do expectations of how far disagreement, rather than consensus, is tolerated within teams. Second, styles of written and oral communication used in academic settings reflect broader cultural patterns. The length of pauses we are comfortable with in discussion, whether interrupting other speakers is legitimate and how animated speakers can be all vary cross-culturally, and differences in discussion styles can be misinterpreted as rudeness or lack of understanding. In written communication, different styles are also favoured in different cultures. One example is the use of citations to other work. In British reports, there is an expectation that the literature and previous research will be reviewed to put findings in context, whereas Chinese scientific reports, for instance, typically focus on the contribution, rather than the background, with the aim of minimizing the 'irrelevant' material for the reader (Cortazzi and Jin 1997: 83). Over long-term collaborations, partners can develop their understanding of these cultural styles, but the time taken to establish good international working relationships is often underestimated.

Conclusion

Few of those working on qualitative health research studies work entirely in isolation. At a minimum, we have to collaborate with research participants from a range of professional and disciplinary backgrounds, and much health research is done in the context of various multi-disciplinary and international collaborations. When qualitative researchers are seen as bringing merely a set of methods (a toolbox of techniques that can be applied to a particular research question), this appears relatively unproblematic: the qualitative component of a project 'adds value' by addressing some issue such as users' views, an exploration of process, or observational description as 'colour' for a report. When qualitative methodology is integrated into a larger project in a more meaningful way, in that researchers bring the theoretical insights and methodological understandings of their disciplines to the research questions, there is a need for more detailed consideration of what each partner expects from the collaboration, and what each expects from the others.

KEY POINTS

- Fruitful collaborative relationships need a considerable investment of time and commitment to establish expectations at the outset over such issues as:
  - the relationships between the different methods used;
  - expected outputs;
  - how the findings will be disseminated;
  - what 'rights' each partner has to the data.
- Epistemological differences between qualitative research approaches and other, more positivist, approaches may pose particular challenges.
- National, disciplinary and professional differences are rarely neutral, and qualitative researchers may have to account for 'differences' more often than those from other backgrounds.

EXERCISE

The European Union is funding a scheme to improve housing and cut the number of excess winter deaths by offering energy efficiency interventions (such as more efficient and affordable heating, improvements in windows) in three partner countries. The interventions are to be evaluated by teams of researchers in each country.

List the disciplines that might need to be involved in a project of this kind and then describe some of the potential benefits and pitfalls that might be encountered. What differences in research perspective might you find and what impact might these have?

One expectation from the evaluation is that findings from the three countries will be compared. What difficulties are you likely to face in developing a protocol suitable for use in all three different countries?

FURTHER READING

There are a number of books on applied medical anthropology that explore the interface between anthropology and public health. One that has chapters on the history of collaboration and a number of interesting case studies is Janes, C.R., Stall, R. and Gifford, S. (1986) *Anthropology and epidemiology: interdisciplinary approaches to the study of health and disease.* Dordrecht: D. Reidel Publishing Company.

There is not a large literature on the process of collaboration, in part because the challenges of working across institutions, disciplines and countries generate often fragile working arrangements that might well be threatened by bringing the conflicts into the public domain. Some examples can be found in the special issue of the journal *Social Policy and Administration* (2000), 34(4), which was on 'The business of research: issues of politics and practice', in which some authors reflect on their experiences of collaborative projects.

10

Writing up Qualitative Work

CHAPTER SUMMARY

Writing is part of the process of doing qualitative research. It is not merely the report of analysis undertaken, but an essential element of that analysis. Qualitative health researchers need to develop their skills in writing for different audiences in order to disseminate their findings not only widely, but also appropriately. This chapter discusses three types of writing typically needed in a qualitative project: articles for health or biomedical journals, writing for social science colleagues, and reports for non–specialist audiences.

Introduction

Writing up a qualitative study can be a very different experience from that of writing up a quantitative one. In part this is because the writing, for most researchers, is part of the analysis. The process of writing (deciding what to include, what order to put it in, how to construct each sentence and paragraph) makes us think in new ways about the data, the connections within the data, and between the data and the broader literature. The very process of writing is part of triggering the 'sociological (or historical, or anthropological) imagination' and identifying the cross-cutting connections that embed your work within the discipline or substantive field of knowledge to which you are contributing. This is why it is good practice to begin writing as soon as possible, rather than as a separate task at the end of the project. This could include writing 'memos' (see Chapter 8) as part of the analysis, writing a reflective diary of the fieldwork process, or descriptive accounts of emerging analysis as the study progresses. Certainly with a substantial piece of writing (such as a PhD thesis) the writing cannot be left to the end; it is an essential *part* of the process of research, rather than a subsequent 'objective' account of that process.

The writing process

Few people find writing easy, and many of us struggle with both getting started and completing the task. Experiences of 'displacement' activities, such as cleaning the house, or filing papers, or making endless cups of coffee to 'get started', are common. We tend to think of these as ways of delaying the real work of writing, but one reassuring perspective incorporates these activities as an essential element *of* writing, rather than a prelude to it. In an interview, Roland Barthes (1985) argued that these practical, or what he called 'ceremonial', aspects of the physical act of writing should not be seen as trivial, and that we should pay attention to the preparatory activities and the materials needed to write. These might include particular settings (do you need to be at a clear desk, or surrounded by files and papers?), routines (do you find it easier to write in long uninterrupted stretches, or in short bursts?) and the tools needed (do you type straight to a PC, or prefer to draft out papers by pen in a notebook first?). On materials, for instance, Barthes discusses the importance of pens to him:

> I would say, for example, that I have an almost obsessive relation to writing instruments. I often switch from one pen to another just for the pleasure of it. I try out new ones … I cannot keep myself from buying them. … In short, I've tried everything … except Bics, with which I feel absolutely no affinity. I would even say, a bit nastily, that there is a 'Bic style', which is really just for churning out copy. … In the end, I always return to fine fountain pens. (Barthes 1985: 178)

Thus, seeming irrelevancies can be taken seriously as part of the task of writing itself, which includes activities such as thinking, planning, and giving yourself opportunities to make imaginative connections within your data. Barthes's descriptions of his writing routines in this interview also suggests some tactics for the difficult point most writers face at times, when there seems no way to begin, or to phrase a particular section. Switching materials may help, in that writing in a notebook if used to typing straight to a screen, or perhaps moving to a new location, may trigger new ideas or ways of thinking about your text.

At a more practical level, the techniques that 'work' to facilitate writing will be personal to you, but there are a number of suggestions that may be useful for getting started and completing the task:

- Draft a detailed structure first, with headings for all the sections you want to include.
- Don't begin at the beginning – it is easiest to write the introduction when you know what is in the body of the text. Start with the section you find easiest or most interesting.
- Think about a specific reader as you write, and about what you are trying to communicate to him or her.
- Try writing your ideas in an everyday, conversational language if you feel defeated by trying to write the 'formal' accounts straight away.
- Regular deadlines. Break large writing tasks into smaller ones, and make sure you have deadlines for each one, by promising drafts or sections to supervisors or co-workers at regular points.

Writing for different audiences

There are a number of potential audiences for any study, particularly in the field of health research, which require tailored writing styles and format. Any or all of the following written outputs might be needed from one study:

- one-page summaries of the key findings for the research participants;
- short paper on the key findings for a practitioners' journal;
- progress reports and final study report for the sponsors;
- executive summary for policy-makers;
- articles for biomedical peer-reviewed journals;
- longer academic article for social science peer-reviewed journals;
- book chapters or a monograph;
- a dissertation or thesis.

Both the content and the style of these papers and reports will be very different, and researchers need a wide range of communication skills to address different audiences in effective ways. Increasingly, researchers are being asked to ensure that potential users of research are informed about outcomes. Users might include practitioners, policy-makers at various levels and voluntary sector groups with an interest in the topic. Participative projects will of course build in considerable attention to communication with research participants throughout the research process, but studies of most kinds will require at least the main results to be disseminated to participants or stakeholders in an appropriate way. Of course, writing for these diverse audiences is not just a matter of writing differently. In some cases we have to *think* differently to write different outputs, putting ourselves in the position of an interviewee, or a practitioner, to think through what the implications of our findings might be. Shifting gear between the different registers needed for these diverse audiences can be difficult, and you may need a gap between writing in different ways.

To illustrate some of these different ways of communicating, we look here at three types of writing you might typically need to do within a qualitative health project: writing for health journals, writing for social science colleagues, and writing for lay audiences.

Writing for health journals

Many qualitative studies in the health field aim to communicate findings not just to other qualitative researchers, but to colleagues from other disciplines or to practitioners. Less lofty aims, such as meeting the institution's needs for good-quality peer-reviewed publications in mainstream journals, are also an incentive for publishing in biomedical and health journals as well as social science ones. In some ways, qualitative findings may be easier to convey to audiences of professionals than complex statistical data, simply because there is an immediacy about accounts of everyday health practices and beliefs that most practitioners can relate to, in terms of their own experiences. Writing for biomedical journals (like any other kind of writing) requires a sensitivity to the audience: what is interesting for practitioners or researchers in other disciplines in your findings and why should they want to read this paper?

The paper needs to be written with the precise readership of the journal in mind, with a clear sense of what is being communicated to them. This will shape the content of the paper, in that you will focus on implications for practice and future research in the area, and perhaps recommendations for those working in the field. Writing up qualitative work for biomedical journals also entails some attention to format and style. Most biomedical journals (look, for instance, at the *British Medical Journal*, or the *Lancet*) expect submitted papers to conform to a standard format designed primarily for quantitative reports, with the following types of headings:

- *Abstract*. Summary of around 150 words, giving purpose of study, setting, methods, main findings and conclusions.
- *Introduction*. Brief overview of aim of study and how this follows from 'what is already known'.
- *Methods*. Methods of data collection and analysis, how sample was selected, description of sample, ethical issues.
- *Results*. Findings of the study, in text or tables.
- *Discussion*. The limitations and implications of the findings in the light of other work, and any recommendations that follow.

Each journal has its own guidelines for authors, often reprinted inside the back cover of each issue of the journal, or available from the journal's or publisher's web page. These will cover issues like the maximum length of an article, how to cite references and whether a structured abstract is needed. Many biomedical journals have adopted the 'Uniform requirements for manuscripts submitted to biomedical journals' (International Committee of Medical Journal Editors 1991), which determine how manuscripts should be prepared (that is, in double-spaced type, using one side of the page, with each section on a new page). These general requirements are also known as the *Vancouver style*, and include requirements for citations and references. In the Vancouver style, references should be cited by inserting an Arabic superscript number in the text when the reference is first used, then listing the full references in number order at the end of the paper.

In addition to these general requirements, most journals have a particular 'house style' that will be more or less constrictive. This influences matters of style such as whether research reports can be written in the first person, whether extensive quotes can be used, whether a detailed methods section is needed, and preferred vocabulary. This can be gauged by reading the qualitative articles published in the journal. There may also be 'checklists' of criteria for qualitative articles submitted to the journal, which are discussed in Chapter 11. It is obviously sensible to write with these in mind where possible, as these may well be used by reviewers who decide whether to recommend your submitted article to the editor for publication.

Of course, many qualitative studies will not fit into this format. It would not be profitable, for instance, to try to force a rich, nuanced description of a healing system from an ethnographic study into a structured format unless there were 'stand-alone' findings that could be separated out and clear messages for the journal readership. Indeed, some claim that the conventional formats developed for reporting the results of quantitative studies are generally too constraining for the adequate reporting of qualitative studies: Matthew Miles and A. Michael Huberman (1994), for instance, argue that structured headings are in general inappropriate because:

> Normally we'd have other expectations for a qualitative report. For example, we might expect a close description of the history, the context, the major actors. . . . We might look for a more 'circular' linkage between research questions, methods, data collection and interim analysis, as each new analysis opened up new leads. (Miles and Huberman 1994: 298)

However, in the health field many qualitative studies are designed to produce 'findings' that can be reported under standard headings. The extract from an abstract in Box 10.1 illustrates the kind of qualitative study that works well for a biomedical journal, in that the authors are able to report their findings under standard headings. This is from a paper by Chris Griffiths and colleagues (Griffiths et al. 2001) published in the *British Medical Journal*.

Box 10.1   Sample abstract from a qualitative study

Influences on hospital admission for asthma in south Asian and white adults: qualitative interview study

Objective: To explore reasons for increased risk of hospital admission among south Asian patients with asthma.

Design: Qualitative interview study using modified critical incident technique and framework analysis. [...]

Main outcome measures: Patients' and health professionals' views on influences on admission, events leading to admission, general practices' organisation and asthma strategies, doctor–patient relationship, and cultural attitudes to asthma.

Results: South Asian and white patients admitted to hospital coped differently with asthma. [...] Patients describing difficulty accessing primary care during asthma exacerbations were registered with practices with weak strategies for asthma care and were often south Asian. [...]

Conclusions: The different ways of coping with asthma exacerbations and accessing primary care may partly explain the increased risk of hospital admission in south Asian patients. [...]

This study, from a multi-disciplinary team (of a sociologist, anthropologist, and primary and secondary care professionals), was clearly designed to address a problem recognizable in clinical practice (the observed increased risk of admission for asthma for some groups in the UK population) and produce findings relevant for practitioners and health promoters working in the area. The data, from interviews, are relatively easy to summarize for readers, and the methodological techniques used (such as framework analysis) can be referred to without too much discussion. However, even for studies like this, where it is possible to divide text up neatly into aims, background, findings and conclusions, the nature of qualitative inquiry does present some particular challenges with this kind of writing. One is the use of quoted material. Whereas a qualitative report may need considerable context and detail to provide credibility and a 'flavour' of the rich, detailed analysis done, biomedical journals may expect brevity and see such material as extraneous. In this example, Griffiths and colleagues have included some brief examples from interviews in the text, and a longer selection in a separate box. Biomedical journals may also require 'quantification' of results, for instance counts of how many respondents had particular attitudes, and rather more transparency about the actual procedures used to analyse the data than is typical in social science journals.

More difficult than these issues of style is the problem of representing the theoretical grounding of the data, and its broader meanings. The space constraints and the 'practical implications' orientation of a biomedical journal mean that it is very difficult to do anything other than hint at what the findings imply for a more conceptual understanding. For this, you will need a more appropriate qualitative format for representing the findings of your study, such as a monograph or a paper for one of the social science journals.

Writing for social science colleagues

There is a huge range of general journals within each of the social science disciplines that publish qualitative studies on health, including those dedicated to the 'medical' sub-disciplines (such as *Medical Anthropology*, *Medical Anthropology Quarterly* and *Sociology of Health and Illness*) and also a number of interdisciplinary journals, such as *Social Science and Medicine* and *Qualitative Health Research*. The various social science disciplines have their own traditions of writing, and each journal has its own favoured styles and approaches. Some publish articles in a more self-consciously 'scientific' style, similar to that in health sciences, in which papers are organized with separate sections on background, literature, methods, findings and discussion and the tone of papers tends to be more 'objective' and neutral, although articles tend to be longer than in the biomedical journals, and include rather more theoretical material. In these, you might be expected to use Vancouver style references. More typically, a social science journal article will have a more narrative style, and will include far more discussion of how the study reported contributes to the discipline. This will require longer background and discussion sections, and the 'findings' section might draw on other literature. The authors need to locate their findings within the theoretical and perhaps methodological debates in the field, and demonstrate not just new empirical data, but how these data extend our conceptual understanding of a problem. Given the importance of situating material within the literature of the discipline, citations to other published work are important, and social science journals usually use what is known as the Harvard style for referencing (as used in this book) in which the author and date of publication are cited in the text, with the full list arranged alphabetically by author at the end of the article.

Some journals explicitly encourage more innovative narrative styles, or expect the material to be organized in an appropriate way for the message of the paper. This could be as a first-person narrative, say, or as a dialogue. The degree to which writing is expected to be reflexive is one key difference, with some qualitative journals encouraging personal, subjective styles in which the author's experiences of doing the research are an essential element of the text. Take, for instance, the opening sentences of one article from the journal *Qualitative Inquiry*, which does encourage a wider range of styles (including, for instance, poems on occasion) than many journals:

Steel doors slam behind me, announcing my progress through the security checks of the detention facility, locally called the 'jail for children', where I am conducting my dissertation research. . . . Combining narrative and ethnographic methods, I hope to describe the relationship between juvenile delinquents and the public institutions charged with the social control of teenagers. . . . But there's a problem: In 2 months of observing . . . I haven't met anyone willing to sign my human subjects' release forms . . . and agree to the interviews I've planned.

Then I meet Clayboy. (VanderStaay 2003: 974)

This, taken from Steven VanderStaay's paper on his research with one teenage drug user in the United States, illustrates the differences between the conventions of biomedical writing and some social science texts. Note that this introduction is in the first person: VanderStaay places himself in the research story from the beginning. He also starts his paper by referring to problems: that two months into his fieldwork, he had failed to find anyone willing to sign the necessary consent forms. This is in stark contrast to the 'post hoc' write-up expected in more scientific styles, in which such problems might be mentioned in the discussion, but are not seen as relevant to the report itself.

The development of a specifically 'scientific' style (relatively plain, neutral, unadorned) separate from a 'literary' style (which uses metaphor and evocative language) is an outcome of post-Enlightenment ideas about science in the West: that it is essentially empirical, in that 'facts speak for themselves', and require transparent language rather than rhetoric to speak for them. Of course, 'scientific' language has its own stylistic persuasiveness. This is achieved through the use of phrases such as 'the findings demonstrate' or 'the study reveals' (which suggest that the facts unearthed 'speak for themselves' without the intervention of the researcher), and the rhetorical use of titles that pose questions to be answered, implying that these will be dealt with authoritatively by the author (Kitzinger 1987; Thorogood 1997). The use of complex tables of numbers and statistical tests and complex technical language are also ways of framing an article as 'scientific' and credible.

So, all writers use 'literary' strategies to increase the credibility of the written report, but in the social sciences it is more common to be explicit about this, and to acknowledge the 'craft' of writing. Kathy Charmaz (1999), for instance, talks about borrowing the strategies of fiction writers to improve writing through providing context for the story, pulling the reader in, recreating mood and adding surprise. Note how VanderStaay, in the extract quoted above, skilfully uses the conventions of story-telling (brief description of a dramatic setting and the quest, setbacks on the way, an unexpected lucky break: 'Then I meet Clayboy') to interest the reader, and also set up some expectations. We understand that, as a researcher trying to complete his dissertation, VanderStaay is perhaps desperate at this point for anyone who will agree, and we understand that his meeting with Clayboy is a pivotal moment, in both his story and that of the research. Rather than a neutral, 'scientific' account of aims and methods, the author has introduced a story in which the 'findings' are clearly going to be closely integrated in and contextualized by the researcher's own role in producing them.

Much qualitative writing for health adopts a scientific style relatively uncritically, in part to establish credibility for audiences familiar with that format. Indeed, there are few examples like that from VanderStaay in the more health-orientated social science journals. In ethnography, in particular, though, there has been considerable debate about writing, and the forms that are appropriate for the textual representation of both the process of researching and descriptions of cultures as the outputs of that research. In part, this follows from a tradition in which personal narratives have had a legitimate place in the writing up of fieldwork, including stories about arriving at the fieldwork site and the challenges faced in learning the language, arranging access and the practicalities of living in the field. Two traditions in anthropology sit in tension: those that stress its 'scientific' status, separate from mere travellers' tales or journalistic anecdotes, and those that recognize subjective experiences as part of establishing the 'authenticity' of the ethnography. The ways in which particular kinds of narrative produce particular possible readings are the subject of debate within the discipline. James Clifford summarizes the various different ways in which ethnographers choose to 'translate experience into text':

> One can 'write up' the results of an individual experience of research. This may generate a realistic account of the unwritten experience of another group or person. One can present this textualization as the outcome of observation, of interpretation, of dialogue. One can construct an ethnography composed of dialogues. One can feature multiple voices, or a single voice. One can portray the other as a stable, essential whole or one can show it to be the product of a narrative of discovery, in specific historical circumstances. (Clifford 1986a: 115)

That these are choices to be debated indicates the focus in ethnography on writing itself as part of the process of representation, rather than merely a tool through which 'findings' are reported for other audiences, but of course Clifford's choices in theory apply to all kinds of writing, not just ethnography. The journal article, or research report, is not a neutral window to the data produced and gathered, but rather a specific narrative that has political effects of its own.

Writing for and disseminating to non-specialist audiences

You may have to feed back results to a number of stakeholders in the research process, such as research participants (interviewees, gatekeepers), potential users of your findings (policy-makers, practitioners) and perhaps wider audiences with the help of the mass media. The incentives for doing this are various, including attempts to influence practice, sharing results with those who helped produce them, and perhaps political purposes, such as generating publicity for your project or department. A common criticism of researchers is that they are poor at communicating their findings in appropriate ways to non-specialist audiences. This is to some extent a matter of style: producing long reports full of technical terms is clearly not an adequate way of informing those who need to use the findings, and preparing summaries of findings for such audiences as research participants means considering some practical aspects of your writing such as:

- *Writing clear, accessible prose.* One way of checking this is to calculate the 'Fog Index' of your writing, as follows:
  - Calculate the average number of words per sentence.
  - Add the percentage of words of three or more syllables to this.

- Multiply by 0.4.

As a rule of thumb, if the result is a Fog Index of more than 12, general readers may find the text difficult. Some word processors have functions that check the readability of text for you. (The sentence that precedes this bullet point scores 24!)

- *Avoid jargon*. We use specialized language and abbreviations as a shorthand to communicate with colleagues, but forget that many of these terms mean nothing (or something rather different!) to non-specialists.

- *Care with vocabulary*. Following on from that, you must be sensitive to ways in which many research users will utilize particular vocabularies. The use of non-discriminatory language is essential in all communication, but you may need to take particular care over language with some groups of users. Most people living with particular illnesses will not want to be described as 'sufferers', for instance, and practitioners will expect their 'technical' vocabularies to be used accurately. Any research on politically sensitive topics, where language may be a site of contestation, will need particular care – see, for instance, Case Study 9.2 on the difficulties of terminology in the Middle East.

- *Appropriate translations*. Some audiences will need specialized translations, for instance into other languages or audio-tape. Below are some suggestions for non-textual forms of feedback, which may be more appropriate for some audiences.

The principles of writing for non-specialist audiences are, though, the same as writing for academic colleagues: you need to think about the reader, what they are likely to want to know, and how to communicate this to them. Research participants and gatekeepers may be interested in issues such as: how typical they were compared with other participants, what is going to happen to the results of the study, whether they will lead to any improvements in practice. The general public (if this is a project likely to attract wider attention) will be primarily interested in the novel or unusual findings, and press releases designed for the mass media will need to focus on what is new or unexpected.

Alternatives to written reports

So far, this chapter has focused on 'writing up' as the most common way in which the findings of qualitative studies are disseminated. It is worth remembering, though, that written output such as reports, journal articles and books may not be the most appropriate ways to represent your research, either because the 'message' or the 'audience' may be best served by other formats. When working in multi-disciplinary settings, textual accounts of the research findings may be particularly difficult for others to access. Here, more visual representations of the findings may be called for, either within traditional prose text or by replacing it on, for instance, posters. Results can be tabulated, pictorial illustrations included, and diagrams can be used to represent connections between findings. Oral presentations of qualitative research are needed for conferences and seminars, and are also a useful way of feeding back results to users such as community groups.

Websites provide a flexible format for reporting and disseminating qualitative findings. It is now relatively easy to create links on web pages to written outputs from projects, but Internet sites also allow more creative use of qualitative data. One good example is the DIPEx (Database of Individual Patients' Experience) project (http://www.dipex.org/EXEC), which is a multi-media website and CD-ROM aimed at patients, carers, health professionals and researchers (Herxheimer et al. 2000). This uses data from a series of qualitative interview studies with patients with serious illnesses to provide information about how people coped with symptoms, found support and decided between treatment options. The main findings from each component qualitative study are summarized under key headings for each disease, and extracts from interviews are available for users to read, listen to or watch on video clips. A searchable website, with links to further information and details on support services, provides an accessible way of making the findings from these studies available to users who might want to look for examples of people who have had similar experiences.

Web-based publishing also offers possibilities for utilizing non-literary forms of communication within academic papers. Hyperlinks, which allow a user of web-based materials to 'click' on a button and move to other points, provide options to include a wealth of other materials alongside the text of the report, such as interview transcripts, links to comments from other authors or to non-textual material. The journal *Sociological Research Online*, for instance, has included recent articles that have hyperlinks to photographs (Thoutenhoofd 1998) and video clips (Lomax and Casey 1998) as part of the paper. Amanda Coffey and colleagues (1996) discuss the particular advantages that hypertext may have for writing qualitative research, given the possibilities it provides for non-linear representations of research outputs, and potentially a more inter-active relationship with readers:

> Many people working with qualitative data, whether they use fieldnotes, interviews, oral history or documentary sources, feel frustrated by the necessity of imposing a single linear order on those materials. It is, after all, part of the rationale of ethnographic and similar approaches that the [researcher] recognizes the complexity of social inter-relatedness. (Coffey et al. 1996: 8.5)

Some practical issues to consider when writing up

Any piece of writing, then, needs to take into account the audience, in terms of what they are likely to want to know and how best to communicate this.

We now turn to some general issues that you might face when writing up qualitative work in the health field.

Authorship

So far, we have assumed that you are the sole author of a qualitative report. This will be true of a research degree thesis, and is still typical in many qualitative social science research projects, but increasingly rare in other health research contexts, where you may be writing with others, or at least with their input. Cultures of authorship differ across disciplines, departments and even individual research teams, with each having their own expectations over such issues as whether team or individual authorship is the norm, or whether supervisors routinely expect to be listed as an author on their students' work. Conflicts over authorship (who is entitled to be named as an author, which order should the names go in?) can be extremely destructive to research teams, and it is good practice to establish responsibilities for writing up material at the beginning of a project. Who will take the lead on which papers? Who will be a contributing author, and who will have rights to edit, or approve, submitted papers?

There are a number of guidelines for establishing rights and responsibilities with regard to authorship. The Vancouver guidelines, discussed above as establishing general requirements for biomedical journals, suggest that the rule of thumb is that each author should be able to defend the paper publicly, but this principle is difficult to put into practice, particularly when reporting studies that have contributors from a number of specialist disciplines. One approach suggests a system more like 'film credits' (Smith 1997), in which the specific contribution of each author is listed (such as research design, drafting the final paper, statistical analysis), and a guarantor named, who can take overall responsibility for a paper. Erol Digusto (1994) has a more complex solution that might be useful for those in larger teams. He suggests a 'points' system, in which all members of a research team award a fixed number of points among the team under headings for each kind of contribution. These are then used to award authorship and position on the authorship list for the list of papers likely to come out of the project in a fair and transparent manner. In practice, at least at the current time, most research teams still make decisions about authorship in an ad hoc manner, and researchers need to develop skills in both explicit negotiations around authorship and writing with colleagues.

Selecting examples and quotes

The amount of quoted material and context you can include will depend on the length of the article and the style of the journal, but in principle you need to include enough for the reader to judge the credibility of your interpretations. However much space you have, though, you will inevitably have to select particular quotes, and perhaps extracts from them, from the entire data set. Choosing particularly evocative or coherent quotes to illustrate findings is fine so long as the content is representative, and the text should indicate whether the extract is typical, or deviant, or perhaps unrepresentatively eloquent. Quotes should be tagged in the text with appropriate identifiers (such as age, gender, or whatever categories are important to the research), or an interview code number if this would breach confidentiality (see below). This both provides context for the reader, and demonstrates that you have not just picked illustrative examples from a small number of interviews.

Even in longer pieces of writing, be wary of 'over-quoting' and expecting your data to do the work that you, as author, should be doing to interpret, explain and make an argument. The quotes are there as *evidence* for your argument. Long articles with many quotes and little text in between look under-analysed, and the reader will not necessarily make the connections between them that you (having done the analysis and the thinking!) will.

Reproducing quotes

In general, quotes in qualitative papers are reproduced verbatim from the interview transcript or fieldwork notes, with the grammar and vocabulary of the original. This can pose a dilemma of balancing readability with veracity, with decisions about how to render, for instance, slang expressions or regional accents. Clearly, some editing always goes on, as a quote reproduced phonetically, with all the pauses and non-verbal noises transcribed, would be almost unreadable, and certainly not give a 'flavour' of the spoken version. Unless reporting the results of a conversation analysis type study (see Chapter 6), most pauses and intonations are not shown, and the spelling (in English-language journals) is standard English, unless the words used by the respondent are dialect or abbreviated. Transcription conventions (see Box 4.2) are used to represent missing text or explanatory words provided by the author.

Quoting material in a different language from the original creates even more acute dilemmas, in deciding whether to reproduce word-for-word translations or attempt to preserve the cultural meanings and nuances of the original. The decision of course depends on what work the quoted material is intended to do within the text. If extracts are there simply to give voice to particular participants, the choice may be to reproduce a 'cultural' translation, which maintains the meaning intended (as far as possible) for a reader using another language. A more ethnographic analysis may require considerable explanatory material in addition to the quote, to alert the reader to relevant context. This might include issues such as how and when similar metaphors are used in this cultural setting, whether this is a relatively formal mode of speaking, whether the particular phrases used are common idioms used rhetorically, or are particular to this respondent.

Maintaining confidentiality for participants

If you have assured participants of confidentiality in final reports, you need to pay particular attention to whether the details of the case studies or intervie-wees you have given could be used to identify them. Code numbers, or perhaps pseudonyms, can be used to tag quotes or extracts from fieldnotes. Pseudonyms for people and places have the advantage of suggesting context, if chosen to reflect the connotations of the original.

Some study designs pose particular problems in terms of confidentiality. Case studies, particularly of atypical or innovative services or settings, may be diffi-cult to disguise, and those in the field are likely to know the site, and possibly even individuals. It is particularly important in these cases to ensure that parti-cipants have read draft reports to ensure they are happy about publication before disseminating more widely.

Making limitations and implications clear

Qualitative research may be an in-depth exploration of one particular setting, or an interview study of a relatively small sample of participants. As we dis-cussed in Chapter 8, the generalizability of these findings is likely to arise from the conceptual transferability of the concepts generated, rather than the statis-tical representativeness of the sample. Readers will expect some comment on both the limitations of how far they can transfer your findings, and what implications the findings have for their own practice, research or theories about the world. Routine or ritualistic accounts of the 'limitations' of qualita-tive work (such as 'this study was based on a small sample') are unhelpful, but it is worth noting the potential threats to generalizability in the study. To take an example from the paper quoted in Box 10.1, note how Griffiths and colleagues (Griffiths et al. 2001) flag up both potential theoretical limitations to their study and the evidence that might mitigate these:

> We are aware of the dangers of stereotyping behaviour in ethnic groups, as well as problems in aggregating groups into classifications which might obscure cultural differ-ences. None the less, distinctions emerged in accounts of south Asians and white patients that are consistent with work. ... (Griffiths et al. 2001: 965)

Other limitations worth discussing are methodological limitations. These can discuss how the methods used and the setting of the research contextualize the data reported. This might include, for instance, explicit reminders for the reader that the study used interview data, and thus concerns *accounts* of phe-nomena, rather than any direct evidence of those phenomena.

As well as noting the limitations, the conclusion section should also draw out the implications for the intended readership. Implications for practice, or for further research, may be 'obvious' to the researchers, who are immersed in the topic and have detailed knowledge, but usually need explicitly marking for the reader.

Telling a story

Finally, a good qualitative paper tells a story. It uses your analytical ideas, related to theory, to take the reader through what you have discovered in your data. In essence, you are not just summarizing your respondents' views, but are presenting your analysis of them. Even for the 'drier', more scientific styles of biomedical journals, it is important for the article to lead the reader through the story you want to tell, rather than leaving them to divine the most salient points, or the new ideas contributed, or the connections between the concepts discussed. The background section should make a good case for why your report is interesting, and how the study you have done meets a need. The findings should flow in the most coherent way possible, rather than be merely a list of 'themes' or points you want to make. A discussion section should draw out the findings, and frame the implications for the reader.

Conclusion

Many researchers find writing a challenge, at least for some kinds of output. Disseminating the findings of qualitative health research increasingly relies on an ability to produce a range of different written texts, and sometimes to think more imaginatively about other formats for reporting. Qualitative health researchers working in multi-disciplinary settings may face a 'double burden' of having to contribute to their discipline (for instance, in writing for mainstream social science journals, or producing monographs) as well as articles for biomedical journals. This is an opportunity, though, as well as a burden. In a practical sense, the outputs of qualitative health research are perhaps more likely to reach those in a position to utilize them than in other qualitative areas of research. In terms of theoretical development, being forced to think through the meaning of research findings from a number of perspectives is a real advantage in ensuring that qualitative data are fully analysed and exploited.

KEY POINTS
- Writing is an essential part of the process of qualitative analysis, and should begin early in the study.
- Qualitative researchers need to develop skills in addressing a range of specific audiences.
- This involves attention to both style and content.

EXERCISE

Take the observations you did for Exercise 2 in Chapter 6. Write up a short account of these in two different styles. Try writing one in the style of a bio-medical journal, and one in a more sociological style. Consider the differences between these two accounts in terms of: vocabulary, structure, whether you wrote in the first person, whether you were focusing on different aspects of your observations.

FURTHER READING

Woods, P. (1999) *Successful writing for qualitative researchers*. London: Routledge. This is a practical text on issues of style and the problems typically faced in writing up qualitative research for social science journals. Includes chapters on both 'standard' and alternative journal formats, with examples largely taken from the sociology of education.

Hall, G.M. (1998) *How to write a paper* (2nd ed.). London: BMJ Books. Taken from short articles in the *British Medical Journal*. Although it does not deal specifically with the demands of writing up qualitative work, this is an excellent guide to the general issues of writing for biomedical journals, with contributions from several journal editors on how to maximize your chances of being published.

11

Reading and Appraising Qualitative Work

CHAPTER SUMMARY

Doing research entails reading the research outputs of others, both to locate our own findings within existing bodies of knowledge, and to develop methodological skills through exposure to as wide a range of material as possible. Reading is a critical activity, in that researchers have to evaluate qualitative work in the context of their own research. In some areas of health research, the formalization of critical appraisal has been advocated, although the application of 'quality checklists' to qualitative research remains contentious.

Introduction

In the previous chapter, we noted that if you are writing for colleagues in the social sciences, demonstrating how your study contributes to the wider discipline or topic is essential. Chapter 8 also touched on the importance of reading for developing the 'social science imagination' that is essential for insightful analysis. This clearly entails a broad reading background: to do good qualitative work requires a familiarity with both the traditional canon of your own discipline, and the more recent relevant work in your topic area. Reading the research outputs of others is, however, not just done to produce the 'Literature

Review' chapter of a thesis, or the background section of a research report. It is an essential element of learning and developing methodological skills. We read journal articles, books and research reports not just to add to our store of empirical knowledge, but to see how others have addressed methodological challenges, or to spark off connections between our own areas of research and those of others. Reading is not a passive task. To read for research involves critical appraisal, in that the aim is to evaluate what you read in terms of the research you have undertaken, or propose to do. This chapter goes on to discuss whether this kind of appraisal can (or should) be formalized for qualitative research, but first we turn to the more general issues of reading in the context of qualitative research.

We bring to reading our own experiences and frameworks of understanding, and re-reading qualitative work often brings different understandings at different points in a research career. There is no single 'true' reading of any text, but a multiple number of possible readings. These change, for instance, over time with the shifting political and social contexts framing particular readings of texts. James Clifford, after discussing the ways in which classic ethnographies now appear (through decades of feminist scholarship) to be 'biased' in terms of their focus on the cultural domains of men, notes:

> In recognising such biases, however, it is well to recall that our own 'full' versions will themselves inevitably appear partial: and if many cultural portrayals now seem more limited than they once did, this is an index of the contingency and historical movement of all readings. No one reads from a neutral or final position. (Clifford 1986b: 18)

He goes on to note that this implies that the notion of identifying 'gaps' in the literature as a rationale for research is a rather limited one. Such gaps will be filled, but in doing so others are revealed, given that there is no possible complete truth that can be read. The 'canon' of literature in whatever field we are researching is not an unchanging corpus of facts to which new findings are accrued, but a shifting field of possible readings. The implications of this for reading for any specific project are twofold. First, it is important not to rely purely on mechanical searches of databases of literature. The use of electronic databases of abstracts (such as PubMed or Medline) is becoming increasingly popular in health research. They do have a very useful function, in generating a number (often a dauntingly large pile!) of useful leads, but this cannot be taken to be the sum total of 'the literature' worth reviewing. Such a comprehensive undertaking is impossible. In doing qualitative work, it is worth reading both widely and imaginatively – including 'classic' works as well as the latest findings in the field, and research reports from outside the narrow field of interest. Readings likely to be of interest to health researchers will come from a number of sources, including books and social science journals (which may not be abstracted on electronic databases), from social sciences research in topics other than health, and also from 'non-research' sources, such as fiction and journalism.

A second implication is that the outcomes of reading are not just a store of new 'facts' to add to our understanding of the topic, but are rather more flexible and contingent. One article might suggest new concepts we can adapt, a monograph might provide a methodological insight, and a novel may spark off a new way of thinking about our data. Re-reading any of these sources will generate different insights at different points in a research career. There is an increasing tendency to look only for the most recent research articles, and to assume that anything published more than ten years ago will have little relevance. Whilst this may be true if working in fast-moving scientific fields, it is worth remembering that human behaviour changes rather slowly. There is often much of value in the 'classic' social science articles and books, and it is usually worth following up original sources where possible, rather than relying on textbook summaries or reviews, as your reading will be framed by the particular problems and concepts that concern you in the context of your own research.

Reading qualitative research, and reading for qualitative research, is as incremental as all other stages of the research process. Reading cannot be restricted to the start of a project, with perhaps a brief check to update the literature review before submitting a paper or handing in a dissertation. Like analysis and writing, it has to be integrated through the whole research process. Early data analysis will generate new ideas and concepts to follow up in the literature, and wide reading throughout the stages of fieldwork and analysis will help develop analytical ideas about the data.

Reading critically

In qualitative research, the result of reading the literature should, then, be rather more than merely summarizing the key points of previous researchers and then listing them, or identifying the empirical 'gaps' in what has been written. Indeed, Harry Wolcott (2002) argues that a traditional literature review may be inappropriate for qualitative research, given that it is merely a device to prove how 'learned' the writer is, and he suggests that we should instead just use literature as and when it is needed within our arguments. However, many research outputs (whether PhD theses or journal articles) will demand something that looks like a literature review. Whether written up as a traditional 'stand-alone' chapter or section, or integrated throughout a piece of writing, there are some specific tasks that the qualitative review should do. For a research degree thesis, one task of the review is still to demonstrate the writer's ability to critically appraise the literature. For all research, though, the key one is to locate your own particular study and its findings in terms of the broader scholarship in your discipline (or disciplines), and you therefore need to *use* the literature to answer a number of questions, such as:

- What theoretical approach(es) does this research question arise from?
- What debates are current within this field, and how does this study contribute to them?
- What areas of consensus are there? That is, what is the received wisdom in the field, what everyone believes to be true?
- What shortcomings in previous scholarship are recognized?

Reading, and writing up your review of the literature, should be a critical exercise that helps a reader of your research see exactly why your study was important (theoretically or practically) and how it builds on previous scholarship, by contributing to debates, undermining 'what is known' or extending understanding. Reviewing the relevant literature for any particular research project requires, then, a 'respectfully critical' approach, which balances an awareness of previous contributions with an appraisal of them. 'Respect' can be particularly difficult in fields like health, where the literature you come across comes from such a wide range of disciplines and theoretical perspectives, some of which may be unfamiliar. Chris Hart, in his book on carrying out literature reviews in the social sciences (Hart 1998), discusses the challenges of coming to this respectful approach when faced with what seem unnecessarily 'difficult' texts:

> ... competence in reading research is not easily acquired. ... It takes time and a willingness to face challenges, acquire new understandings and have sufficient openness of mind to appreciate that there are other views of the world. ... This means not categorizing the text using prejudicial perceptions of the study discipline, but instead placing the research in the context of norms of the discipline. (Hart 1998: 11)

Critical appraisal involves, then, understanding research outputs in their own terms, and persevering with what can seem at first sight to be jargon-filled or overly complex accounts from unfamiliar fields. In addition to being 'respectful', though, reading for research needs to be evaluative, in identifying both the contributions and the shortcomings of what has gone before. Evaluation entails appraising qualitative research in its own terms (Was the methodological approach appropriate for the question? Is the analysis credible?) and also in terms of broader questions about its contribution to knowledge.

Appraising empirical work: are criteria possible?

We all evaluate or appraise work when we read it, in deciding whether it is well written, useful, credible or flawed. This appraisal is done for particular purposes. Journal reviewers are judging whether the manuscript is appropriate for the journal readership, meets certain (sometimes formal) criteria of 'sound' research and is written in an acceptable style. PhD students judge whether particular articles are relevant for their topic or important to the field they are studying. One question that has divided qualitative researchers is whether we should try to formalize these implicit criteria that are used to make these kinds of appraisals. A key problem, of course, is that the different epistemological approaches, theoretical starting points and methodological choices made by qualitative researchers would imply rather different criteria, if we were being 'respectful' and judging qualitative outputs in their own terms. Is it possible to come to any consensus about what constitutes 'quality' in written accounts of qualitative research?

The increasing interest in using the findings from qualitative research in health has generated substantial interest in trying to do just this. The incentives for attempting what seems to be an impossible task come from a number of directions:

- *The growing interest in 'evidence-based health care'.* In the field of health, there has been a powerful movement for using research evidence to inform both policy and clinical decision-making (Sackett et al. 1996; Gray 1997). If qualitative findings are to be included in an 'evidence base' (Green and Britten 1998), it has been argued, we need some way of appraising the quality of evidence from these studies in order to synthesize empirical findings (Mays et al. 2001).
- *The increasing acceptability of qualitative work to biomedical journal editors.* Given the lack of training in social sciences methodology of many journal editors and reviewers, there has been a demand for criteria to help them make decisions about the quality of articles submitted for publication.
- *Interest in multi-disciplinary studies in health care.* When working across disciplines, it can be helpful for those from non-social science traditions to have guidelines for reading unfamiliar types of literature, to suggest how they might evaluate the validity and usefulness of contributions that use unfamiliar methodologies.

Over the last decade, a number of 'checklists' for appraising qualitative empirical articles have been generated, in part to meet the needs identified above (see, for instance, Boulton et al. 1996; Popay et al. 1998; Mays and Pope 1999; Blaxter 2000). The use of 'checklists' to appraise qualitative work does raise a number of questions:

- Given the range of designs and approaches in qualitative research, is it desirable to try to reach a consensus on what the 'criteria of quality' should be?
- If it is desirable, is it possible to 'operationalize' the procedures readers use when judging quality? That is, is it possible to reify the elements of quality in such a way that they can be clearly described as 'quality criteria' for readers to evaluate the research, rather than merely what has been included in the report? This is essentially a question about the *validity* of checklists.
- If it is desirable and possible, how far would different readers agree on whether criteria had been met or not? That is, is it possible to develop *reliable* checklists, which could be used to reach a consensus on the quality of an empirical report of qualitative work?

In general terms, it is probably impossible to develop a consensus view on what the criteria of good quality should be for all empirical qualitative work. The different epistemological starting points, methodological approaches and disciplinary traditions would all imply rather different evaluations of what 'good research' would look like. However, most checklists are not aiming to identify criteria for 'quality' per se, but rather criteria for *appropriateness* for particular uses. These uses might include publication in a particular journal, or perhaps inclusion in a literature review of the qualitative evidence on a particular topic. For use in a literature review, the questions around the reliability of guidelines could be addressed through using more than one reviewer, so that the degree of consensus on how far each paper considered met the criteria could be measured.

Appraisal criteria

The various checklists that have been developed cover a number of common issues, although obviously there are differences reflecting the different functions they were designed to perform. Mildred Blaxter, on behalf of the UK Medical Sociology Group (Blaxter 2000), developed the list that is summarized in Box 11.1, for circulation to medical journal editors to assist them in appraising qualitative work. They were not designed to be comprehensive or exhaustive, and not all researchers would agree on these as markers of quality, but they do cover the main topics that readers using literature to inform a review for evidence, or judging the appropriateness of findings for a general health care audience, might need to consider.

Many of the criteria summarized in Box 11.1 were discussed in Chapter 8 as elements of rigorous analysis. They are, at this level, not particularly contentious − especially if it is remembered that they are aiming not to legislate for what qualitative work *should* look like, but merely to highlight questions that readers of particular sorts (such as editors of biomedical journals, or reviewers carrying out a literature review for policy-making) might want to consider in judging whether the research has been conducted and reported appropriately. However, the use of such 'checklists' has prompted debate about what is 'lost' from the qualitative tradition in attempting to formalize good practice guidelines in this way.

A first criticism is that they do not reflect current practice. Mary Boulton and colleagues (Boulton et al. 1996) searched for all the qualitative reports in five years of publishing from seven medical journals, and found 70 examples that had used qualitative methods of data collection and analysis. Of these, they found that the majority appropriately used qualitative methods for the research question, but fewer would meet other quality criteria. Using a similar list to that summarized in Box 11.1, Boulton and colleagues found that about half of the papers met most of the criteria, but that there were typically shortcomings over such criteria as: providing sufficient original material to satisfy the reader

Box 11.1   Some criteria for the evaluation of qualitative research papers

Criteria	Examples
Research design: Are the methods appropriate for the research question?	Does the research seek to understand processes or structures, or illuminate subjective experiences or meanings?
Theory: Is the connection to an existing body of knowledge or theory clear?	Is there adequate reference to the literature? Does the work cohere with, or critically address, existing theory?
Transparency of procedures: Are there clear accounts of the sampling strategy, data collection and analysis?	Is the selection of cases or participants theoretically justified?
Has the relationship between fieldworkers and participants been considered?	How did research participants perceive the research?
Was data collection and record-keeping systematic?	Were careful records kept? Were full records or transcripts used, if appropriate?
Analysis: Is reference made to acceptable procedures for analysis?	Is it clear how analysis was done?
How systematic was the analysis?	Has reliability been considered?
Is there adequate discussion of how themes, concepts or categories were derived from the data?	What steps were taken to guard against selectivity in the use of data?
Is there adequate discussion of the evidence for and against the researcher's arguments?	Are negative data given? Has there been a search for 'deviant cases'?
Presentation: Is the research clearly contextualized?	Is there relevant information about the settings and participants? Are the cases or variables integrated into their social context, rather than abstracted and decontextualized?
Are the data presented systematically?	Are quotations, fieldnotes, etc., identified such that the reader can judge the range of evidence being used?
Is there a clear distinction between data and interpretation?	Do the conclusions follow from the data?
Is the author's own position clearly stated?	Has the impact of this on the research been explored?
Value: Are the results credible and appropriate?	Do they address the research question? Are they plausible and coherent? Are they important, either theoretically or practically?
Ethics: Have ethical issues been adequately considered?	Has the issue of confidentiality been considered? Have the consequences of the work been considered?

about the relationship between data and interpretation, steps to improve validity of the analysis, steps to improve reliability, and the processes of data analysis.

A second possible criticism of the application of checklists is that the more interpretative elements of analysis, which, arguably, result in interesting and more conceptually satisfying findings, are rather difficult to describe. Boulton and colleagues note that even the more mundane processes of analysis (how coding schemes were developed and applied, for instance) can be very difficult to describe, but they argue that this is an essential element of providing credible evidence.

Third, as we noted in Chapter 8, few of the 'classic' qualitative studies that have had an impact on the field of health and illness, and reported in monographs or social science journals, would meet the kinds of criteria suggested above. Boulton and colleagues consider the concern that quality criteria would 'inhibit more purely creative and imaginative uses of qualitative methods . . . and rule governed research would less frequently produce the startling narrative found in the works of, say, Goffman or Becker' (Boulton et al. 1996: 178). However, they find this an unconvincing argument, at least applied to the kinds of qualitative research reported in health journals. As they note, little of the work they reviewed 'aspired to such creative use of the qualitative method', and on balance they argue that there are advantages in moving towards consensus and transparency around how we judge the quality of qualitative reports.

Finally, a practical shortcoming of criteria checklists is that adequate space for addressing all the issues covered in guidelines (locating the study in a body of theory, context, details of the analysis, reflexivity) is rarely available in a medical journal, which might provide 2000 words. One response some journals have to this problem is to provide longer web-based versions, in which further details of, say, analysis procedures can be discussed.

A more fundamental problem with guidelines is perhaps the range of qualitative methodological approaches that generate useful findings for health, and the danger that producing checklists for journals to use will restrict the range of research undertaken, as being able to publish findings is one factor in deciding how and what to research. There are resulting problems with researchers 'writing to the guidelines' in rather unreflective and routine ways. It is not uncommon, for instance, to come across such claims in medical journal qualitative papers as 'Reliability was maximized by using two people to code the data' or 'Grounded theory was used to analyse the data'. Such sentences tell the reader little (How did the two coders develop their conceptual coding scheme from their discussions? In what ways did a grounded theory approach inform the design and analysis of the study?), and there is a sense that they have been inserted to 'tick the box on a checklist' and maximize the chance of publication, rather than adopted to maximize the validity of the analysis.

It could also be noted that guidelines might work relatively well for small-scale interview studies that have been analysed using thematic content analysis, which do form the bulk of qualitative contributions to medical journals (Boulton et al. 1996), but are perhaps considerably less useful for other study designs (such as ethnographic studies, complex action research projects), or other analytical approaches (such as conversation analysis, the findings from a 'saturated' grounded theory study). Ethnographers, in particular, have debated the issue of criteria for qualitative writing, and in general have been less accepting of the 'checklist' approach than qualitative health service researchers.

Criteria in ethnography

Reviewing the various positions in the debate on 'criteria' for appraisal in ethnography, Martyn Hammersley (1992b: 57–68) outlines three possible positions, which could be summarized as:

1   Given that qualitative research does not start from a positivist position, there can be no privileged position from which to assess the 'truth' or trustworthiness of a particular account. Therefore, the idea of quality criteria is a logical impossibility.
2   Ethnography, in claiming to produce 'scientific' findings, should be judged in terms of the same criteria that any research is judged by.
3   Ethnography, as an alternative paradigm, and as drawing on non-positivistic epistemological underpinnings, requires a particular set of criteria for judging quality.

Rejecting the first two, on the grounds that the relativism of (1) would undercut the basis of rational discussion and that the kinds of models implied by (2) are those of quantitative research, with concepts that are inadequate for judging qualitative, non-experimental studies, he develops some suggestions under (3). His argument for the need for criteria is that he believes that the aim of ethnographic research should be to 'provide information that is both true and relevant to some legitimate public concern' (Hammersley 1992b: 68), and that criteria should therefore relate to both validity and relevance. On the first, validity (the 'truth' of the account), he argues that ethnographic writing should be judged in terms of plausibility and credibility. The reader essentially asks: are the findings plausible, and is there sufficient evidence provided to make the claims made credible? Clearly, the less plausible findings are (in that they are, say, out of line with our expectations or the accepted consensus), the more evidence a reader will need to be convinced of their credibility. Here, Hammersley demonstrates the need for sensitivity to the needs of different audiences: to make findings credible for, say, general practitioners compared with a patients' organization, we would probably need to include different levels of detail on the various sorts of evidence from the study. His second criterion is 'relevance', in terms of the importance of the topic and how it contributes to the literature. These criteria have considerable appeal to areas such as health care ethnography, where (multi-disciplinary) audiences are generally demanding of both credibility and relevance.

Hammersley stays at the level of the 'evidence' in discussing criteria for assessing the quality of ethnographic work in terms of what it contributes. Others have attempted to integrate the aesthetic criteria that in practice are a large element of our reaction to a particular piece of work. In judging whether a piece of research is credible or not, we are as likely to be persuaded by writing style and rhetorical skill as any more 'objective' notions of the strength of evidence. Laurel Richardson (2000), in a bid to combine both 'scientific' and 'literary' criteria for judging qualitative work, outlines five criteria that she uses when reviewing papers and monographs:

- substantive contribution to our understanding of social life;
- aesthetic merit;
- reflexivity, including an account of how the text came to be written, whether there is enough about the author to judge their point of view and ethical issues;
- impact – does it have an emotional and intellectual impact on the reader?
- expression of a reality – is it credible?

This attempts to see the aims of writing up as rather broader than merely adding (valid) empirical evidence to what is known about a topic. Other ethnographic writers go further, with arguments under Hammersley's first position: that it is impossible to come up with 'objective' criteria for appraising qualitative research. Arthur Bochner (2000), for instance, argues that the obsession with criteria is evidence of 'our insecurities about our scientific stature', and unwillingness to admit that the phenomena that qualitative researchers study are 'messy, complicated, uncertain and soft'. Criteria focus the researcher towards rigour rather than imagination, and questions of 'truth' rather than possibility. Bochner is not advocating an 'anything goes' approach, but rather a concern with the narratives that, for him, are the core of research, and the unique contribution of ethnography. Thus, in appraising writing, he reports six elements of narratives that are important for him. These link experiences and meanings, and bring in the imaginative and poetic aspects of the writing. These are summarized in Box 11.2.

Box 11.2   Bochner's criteria for judging 'poetic social science'

- Detail, of the commonplace, of feelings as well as facts.
- Narratives that are structurally complex and take account of time as it is experienced.
- A sense of the author, their subjectivity and 'emotional credibility'.
- Stories that tell about believable journeys through the life course.
- Ethical self-consciousness: respect for others in the field, and for the moral dimensions of the story.
- A story that moves the reader at an emotional as well as a rational level.

Source: Adapted from Bochner (2000).

Reading qualitative research for health, we are often drawn to the criteria of rigour summarized in Box 11.1, for these are framed in ways that are familiar to colleagues from other disciplines, and orientated towards producing 'evidence' that is 'useful' (because it is credible) for practice. However, Bochner's alternative suggestions are a reminder that what qualitative research often aims to provide is not evidence, but insight, and not credibility, but possibility. Reading widely, and appraising in ways appropriate to both our disparate research needs and the aims of the writer, is the best way of ensuring that our own research can contribute in terms of both evidence and insight.

Conclusion

The debate about criteria for evaluating qualitative research centres on a division about what research is for: whether to add to an evidence base, in which case we need criteria in order to judge the validity and usefulness of that evidence, or whether to provide a more unique, qualitative contribution to our understanding of health, which involves insightful understanding of concepts of health and illness in terms of people's lived experience. The former perspective is perhaps typical of qualitative health services research, whereas the latter is debated most heatedly in ethnography. Most researchers shift between the two perspectives, and of course utilize the arguments of each rhetorically at times, in order to persuade particular audiences of the value of their methods.

In conclusion, there is a now a huge qualitative health research literature, and an even wider range of potentially useful readings for qualitative health researchers. In this chapter we have suggested that doing 'good' qualitative research in health involves familiarity with this literature, and a respectful appraisal of it in terms of how past scholarship has contributed to the questions we ask and how we consider answering them. A broad reading experience is perhaps an essential precondition for contributing your own insights to the field of qualitative research in health.

KEY POINTS
- Doing good qualitative work requires broad reading.
- Reading for research should be both respectful and critical.
- There is considerable debate as to whether criteria for assessing the quality of qualitative work are possible or desirable.

EXERCISE

Choose two qualitative articles you have enjoyed, one from a social science journal and one from a biomedical journal. Assess them both in terms first of the criteria summarized in Box 11.1 and then in Box 11.2. Did the 'scores' reflect your own views of the usefulness, quality or contribution of the articles? If possible, compare your evaluations with those of a colleague. How reliable are such guidelines?

FURTHER READING

Clifford, J. and Marcus, G. (1986) *Writing culture: the poetics and politics of ethnography.* Berkeley: University of California Press. A collection of essays on the topic of representation in ethnography, which explore from a number of perspectives the status of texts and authors. Interesting reading for those looking to challenge the ways in which they read qualitative products, and look at texts in their literary, political and ethical contexts.

Hart, C. (1998) *Doing a literature review: releasing the social science research imagination.* London: Sage. Aimed at postgraduate students needing to do a literature review for a dissertation or thesis, but this is also an excellent text for other researchers on what the aims of reading should be and how we can communicate material gathered from reviews.

References

Adamson, C. (1997) 'Existential and clinical uncertainty in the medical encounter: an idiographic account of an illness trajectory defined by inflammatory bowel disease and avascular necrosis', *Sociology of Health and Illness*, 19: 133–59.

Agar, M.H. (1980) *The professional stranger: an informal introduction to ethnography*. San Diego: Academic Press.

Andrews, L., Stocking, C., Krizek, T., et al. (1997) 'An alternative strategy for studying adverse events in medical care', *Lancet*, 349: 309–13.

Annandale, E. (1998) *The sociology of health and medicine*. London: Polity.

Annett, H. and Rifkin, S. (1995) *Guidelines for rapid participatory appraisals to assess community health needs*. Geneva: World Health Organization.

Armstrong, D. (1986) 'The invention of infant mortality', *Sociology of Health and Illness*, 8: 211–32.

ASA (Association of Social Anthropologists) (1987) *Ethical guidelines for good practice*. London: Association of Social Anthropologists.

Atkinson, P. (1995) *Medical talk and medical work: the liturgy of the clinic*. London: Sage.

Backhouse, G. (2002) 'How preserving confidentiality in qualitative health research can be compatible with preserving data for future use', *Medical Sociology News*, 28(2): 32–5.

Baker, R. and Hinton, R. (1999) 'Do focus groups facilitate meaningful participation in social research?', in R. Barbour and J. Kitzinger (eds), *Developing focus group research: politics, theory and practice*. London: Sage, pp. 79–98.

Barthes, R. (1985) 'An almost obsessive relation to writing instruments', in *The grain of the voice*. New York: Hill & Wang, pp. 177–82.

Basch, C.E. (1987) 'Focus group interview: an underutilized research technique for improving theory and practice in health education', *Health Education Quarterly*, 14: 411–48.

Baum, F. (1995) 'Researching public health: behind the qualitative-quantitative methodological debate', *Social Science and Medicine*, 40: 459–68.

Beauchamp, T.L. and Childress, J.F. (1983) *Principles of biomedical ethics* (2nd ed.). Oxford: Oxford University Press.

Becker, H. (1967) 'Whose side are we on?', *Social Problems*, 14: 239–47.

Becker, H. and Geer, B. (1957) 'Participant observation and interviewing: a comparison', *Human Organization*, 16: 28–32.

Becker, M.H. (1974) 'The health belief model and personal health behaviour', *Health Education Monographs*, 2: 324–508.

Beckerleg, S., Lewando-Hundt, G.A., Borkan, J.M., Abu Saad, K.J. and Belmaker, I. (1997) 'Eliciting local voices using natural group interviews', *Anthropology and Medicine*, 4: 273–88.

Bendelow, G. (1993) 'Using visual imagery to analyse gender differences in perception of pain', in C. Renzetti and R. Lee (eds), *Researching sensitive subjects*. London: Sage, pp. 212–229.

Berger, P.L. and Luckman, T. (1967) *The social construction of reality*. Harmondsworth: Penguin.

Black, N. (1994) 'Why we need qualitative research', *Journal of Epidemiology and Community Health*, 48: 425–6.

Blaxter, M. (2000) 'Criteria for qualitative research', *Medical Sociology News*, 26: 34–7.

Bloor, M., Frankland, J., Thomas, M. and Robson, K. (2001) *Focus groups in social research*. London: Sage.

Bochner, A.P. (2000) 'Criteria against ourselves', *Qualitative Inquiry*, 6: 266–72.

Bond, S. and Bond, J. (1982) 'A Delphi study of clinical nursing research priorities', *Journal of Advanced Nursing*, 7: 565–75.

Boulton, M., Fitzpatrick, R. and Swinburne, C. (1996) 'Qualitative research in health care. II. A structured review and evaluation of studies', *Journal of Evaluation in Clinical Practice*, 2: 171–9.

Bowden, A., Fox-Rushby, J.A., Nyandieka, L. and Wanjau, J. (2002) 'Methods for pre-testing and piloting survey questions: illustrations from the KENQOL survey of health-related quality of life', *Health Policy and Planning*, 17: 322–30.

Bowker, G.C. and Star, S.L. (1999) *Sorting things out: classification and its consequences*. Cambridge, MA: MIT Press.

Bowler, I. (1995) 'Further notes on record taking and making in maternity care: the case of south Asian descent women', *Sociological Review*, 43: 36–51.

Britten, N., Campbell, R., Pope, C., Donovan, J., Morgan, M. and Pill, R. (2002) 'Using meta-ethnography to synthesise qualitative research: a worked example', *Journal of Health Services Research and Policy*, 7: 209–15.

Bryman, A. (1988) *Quantity and quality in social research*. London: Routledge.

BSA (British Sociological Association) (1992) 'BSA statement of ethical practice', *Sociology*, 26: 703–7.

Bulmer, M. (1982) 'The research ethics of pseudo-patient studies: a new look at the merits of covert ethnographic methods', *Sociological Review*, 30: 627–46.

Bulmer, M. (1984) *Sociological research methods: an introduction* (2nd ed.). Basingstoke: Macmillan.

Burghart, R. (1993) 'His Lordship at the Cobblers' well', in M. Hobart (ed.), *An anthropological critique of development*. London: Routledge, pp. 77–99.

Bury, M. (1986) 'Social constructionism and the development of medical sociology', *Sociology of Health and Illness*, 8: 137–69.

Busby, H. (2000) 'Writing about health and sickness: an analysis of contemporary autobiographical writing from the British Mass-Observation Archive', *Sociological Research Online*, 5(2) (http://www.socresonline.org.uk/5/2/busby.html).

Butler, J. (1990) *Gender trouble: feminism and the subversion of identity*. New York: Routledge.

Cassell, J. (1980) 'Ethical principles for conducting fieldwork', *American Anthropologist*, 82: 28–41.

Chard, J.A., Lilford, R.J. and Court, B.V. (1997) 'Qualitative medical sociology: what are its crowning achievements?', *Journal of the Royal Society of Medicine*, 90: 604–9.

Charmaz, K. (1999) 'Stories of suffering: subjective tales and research narratives', *Qualitative Health Research*, 9: 362–82.

CIOMS (1991) *Ethics and epidemiology: international guidelines (Proceedings of the XXVth CIOMS Conference, 1990, Geneva)*. Geneva: Council for International Organizations of Medical Science.

Clifford, J. (1986a) 'On ethnographic allegory', in J. Clifford and G. Marcus (eds), *Writing culture: the poetics and politics of ethnography*. Berkeley: University of California Press, pp. 98–121.

Clifford, J. (1986b) 'Introduction: partial truths', in J. Clifford and G. Marcus (eds), *Writing culture: the poetics and politics of ethnography*. Berkeley: University of California Press, pp. 1–26.

Coffey, A., Holbrook, B. and Atkinson, P. (1996) 'Qualitative data analysis: technologies and representations', *Sociological Research Online*, 1(1) (http://www.socresonline.org.uk/socresonline/1/1/4.html).

Coreil, J. (1995) 'Group interview methods in community health research', *Medical Anthropology*, 16: 193–210.

Cornwell, J. (1984) *Hard earned lives: accounts of health and illness from East London*. London: Tavistock.

Cortazzi, M. and Jin, L. (1997) 'Communication for learning across cultures', in D. McNamara and R. Harris (eds), *Overseas students in higher education: issues in teaching and learning*. London: Routledge, pp. 76–90.

Cosby, N., Kelly, J.M. and Shaefer, P. (1986) 'Citizens' panels: a new approach to citizen participation', *Public Administration Review*, 46: 170–8.

Craig, G., Corden, A. and Thornton, P. (2000) *Safety in social research* (Social Research Update 29). Guildford: University of Surrey.

Danziger, R. (1998) 'HIV testing for HIV prevention: a comparative analysis of policies in Britain, Hungary and Sweden', *AIDS Care*, 10: 563–70.

Davison, C., Davey Smith, G. and Frankel, S. (1991) 'Lay epidemiology and the prevention paradox: the implications of coronary candidacy for health education', *Sociology of Health and Illness*, 13: 1–19.

Denzin, N.K. (1971) 'The logic of naturalistic inquiry', *Social Forces*, 50: 166–82.

Denzin, N.K. (1989a) *Interpretative biography* (Qualitative Research Methods Series 17). Newbury Park, CA: Sage.

Denzin, N.K. (1989b) 'Strategies of multiple triangulation', in *The research act: a theoretical introduction* (3rd ed.). Englewood Cliffs, NJ: Prentice-Hall, pp. 234–47.

Denzin, N.K. (1994) 'The art and politics of interpretation', in N.K. Denzin and Y.S. Lincoln (eds), *Handbook of qualitative research*. London: Sage, pp. 500–15.

Denzin, N.K. and Lincoln, Y.S. (1998) 'Introduction: entering the field of qualitative research', in N.K. Denzin and Y.S. Lincoln (eds), *Strategies of qualitative inquiry*. Thousand Oaks, CA: Sage, pp. 1–34.

Desvouges, W.H. and Smith, V.K. (1988) 'Focus groups and risk communication: the "science" of listening to data', *Risk Analysis*, 8: 479–84.

Dexter, L.A. (1970) *Elite and specialized interviewing*. Evanston, IL: Northwestern University Press.

DiGiacomo, S. (1999) 'Can there be a cultural epidemiology?', *Medical Anthropology Quarterly*, 13: 436–57.

Digusto, E. (1994) 'Equity in authorship: a strategy for assigning credit when publishing', *Social Science and Medicine*, 38: 55–8.

DOH (Department of Health) (2001) *Governance arrangements for NHS Research Ethics Committees*. London: DOH.

Draper, A., Green, J. and Dowler, E. (2002) *Public perceptions of BSE and CJD risk in Europe. Final Report for Task 1: Inter-country results and comparisons.* Geneva: WHO.

Edwards, R. (1990) 'Connecting method and epistemology: a white woman interviewing black women', *Women's Studies International Forum,* 13: 477–90.

Ehrich, K. (2001) 'It could be you', *Medical Sociology News,* 27: 23–4.

Esposito, N. (2001) 'From meaning to meaning: the influence of translation techniques on non-English focus group research', *Qualitative Health Research,* 11: 568–79.

Evans, M., Stoddart, H., Condon, L., Freeman, E., Grizzell, M. and Mullen, R. (2001) 'Parents' perspectives on the MMR immunisation: a focus group study', *British Journal of General Practice,* 51: 904–10.

Fahim, H. (ed.) (1982) *Indigenous anthropology in non-western countries.* Durham, NC: Carolina Academic Press.

Fielding, N. (1994) 'Getting into computer-aided qualitative data analysis', *ESRC Data Archive Bulletin* (Sept.).

Fielding, N. (1995) 'Choosing the right qualitative software package', *ESRC Data Archive Bulletin,* 54 (May).

Finch, J. (1984) ' "It's great to have someone to talk to": ethics and politics of interviewing women', in C. Bell and H. Roberts (eds), *Social researching: politics, problems and practice.* London: Routledge, pp. 70–87.

Fineman, N. (1991) 'The social construction of noncompliance: a study of health care and social service providers in everyday practice', *Sociology of Health and Illness,* 13: 354–75.

Gabbay, J. (1982) 'Asthma attacked?', in P. Wright and A. Treacher (eds), *The problems of medical knowledge: examining the social construction of medicine.* Edinburgh: Edinburgh University Press, pp. 23–48.

Gallagher, M., Hares, T., Spencer, J., Bradshaw, C. and Webb, I. (1993) 'The Nominal Group Technique: a research tool for general practice?', *Family Practice,* 10: 76–81.

Garfinkel, H. (1967) *Studies in ethnomethodology.* Englewood Cliffs, NJ: Prentice-Hall.

Gillon, R. (ed.) (1994) *Principles of health care ethics.* Chichester: John Wiley.

Glaser, B. and Strauss, A. (1967) *The discovery of grounded theory: strategies for qualitative research.* Chicago: Aldine.

Godin, B. and Gingras, Y. (2000) 'Impact of collaborative work on academic science', *Science and Public Policy,* 27: 65–73.

Goffman, E. (1961) *Asylums: essays on the social situation of mental patients and other inmates.* New York: Doubleday.

Goffman, E. (1963) *Stigma: notes on the management of a spoiled identity.* Englewood Cliffs, NJ: Prentice-Hall.

Gold, R.L. (1958) 'Roles in sociological field observation', *Social Forces,* 36: 217–23.

Gorard, S. (2002) *Ethics and equity: pursuing the perspectives of non-participants* (Social Research Update 39). Guildford: University of Surrey.

Gordon, D. (1988) 'Tenacious assumptions in Western medicine', in M. Lock and D. Gordon (eds), *Biomedicine examined.* Dordrecht: Kluwer Academic Publishers, pp. 19–56.

Graham, H. (1987) 'Women's smoking and family health', *Social Science and Medicine,* 25: 47–56.

Gray, J.A.M. (1997) *Evidence based health care: how to make health policy and management decisions.* Edinburgh: Churchill Livingstone.

Green, J. (1993a) 'The views of single handed general practitioners: a qualitative study', *British Medical Journal*, 307: 607–10.

Green, J. (1993b) *The problems faced by single handed general practitioners: study report.* London: Department of General Practice, UMDS.

Green, J. (1997) *Risk and misfortune.* London: UCL Press.

Green, J. (1999) 'From accidents to risk: public health and preventable injury', *Health, Risk and Society*, 1: 25–39.

Green, J. and Britten, N. (1998) 'Qualitative research and evidence based medicine', *British Medical Journal*, 316: 1230–4.

Green, J. and Hart, L. (1999) 'The impact of context on data', in R. Barbour and J. Kitzinger (eds), *Developing focus group research: politics, theory and practice.* London: Sage, pp. 21–35.

Green, J., Free, C. and Newman, T. (2002a) *Bilingual children/monolingual parents.* Final Report for ESRC, award number R000223433.

Green, J., Siddall, H. and Murdoch, I. (2002b) 'Learning to live with glaucoma: a qualitative study of diagnosis and the impact of sight loss', *Social Science and Medicine*, 55: 257–67.

Green, J., Draper, A. and Dowler, E. (2003) 'Short cuts to safety: risk and "rules of thumb" in accounts of food choice', *Health, Risk and Society*, 5: 33–52.

Greenhalgh, T. and Hurwitz, B. (1998) *Narrative based medicine: dialogue and discourse in clinical practice.* London: BMJ Books.

Griffiths, C., Kaur, G., Gantley, M., Feder, G., Hillier, S., Goddard, J. and Packe, G. (2001) 'Influences on hospital admission for asthma in south Asian and white adults: qualitative interview study', *British Medical Journal*, 323: 962–6.

Grinyer, A. (2002) *The anonymity of research participants: assumptions, ethics and practicalities* (Social Research Update 36). Guildford: University of Surrey.

Hakim, C. (1982) *Secondary analysis in social research.* London: Allen & Unwin.

Hammersley, M. (1992a) 'So, what are case studies?', in *What's wrong with ethnography?* London: Routledge, pp. 183–200.

Hammersley, M. (1992b) 'By what criteria should ethnographic work be judged?', in *What's wrong with ethnography?* London: Routledge, pp. 57–82.

Hammersley, M. and Atkinson, P. (1983) *Ethnography: principles in practice.* London: Routledge.

Haraway, D. (1991) *Simians, cyborgs, and women: the re-invention of nature.* New York: Routledge.

Hardey, M. (1999) 'Doctor in the house: the internet as a source of lay health knowledge and the challenge to expertise', *Sociology of Health and Illness*, 21: 820–35.

Harding, S. (1986) *The science question in feminism.* Milton Keynes: Open University Press.

Harrison, B. (1996) 'Every picture "tells a story": uses of the visual in sociological research', in E.S. Lyon and J. Busfield (eds), *Methodological imaginations.* London: Macmillan, pp. 75–94.

Hart, C. (1998) *Doing a literature review: releasing the social science research imagination.* London: Sage.

Hart, E. and Bond, M. (1995) *Action research for health and social care: a guide to practice.* Buckingham: Open University Press.

Harvey, L. (1990) *Critical social research.* London: Unwin Hyman.

HCPO (Hopi Cultural Preservation Office) (2001) *HCPO policy and research* (http://www.nau.edu/~hcpo-p/hcpo/index.html).

Helman, C.G. (1978) 'Feed a cold, starve a fever', *Culture, Medicine and Psychiatry*, 2: 107–37.

Helman, C.G. (1984) *Culture, health and illness*. Bristol: Wright.

Henderson, L., Kitzinger, J. and Green, J. (2000) 'Representing infant feeding: content analysis of British media portrayals of bottle feeding and breast feeding', *British Medical Journal*, 321: 1196–8.

Henderson, L.J. (1935) 'Physician and patient as a social system', *New England Journal of Medicine*, 212: 819–23.

Herxheimer, A., McPherson, A., Miller, R., Shepperd, S., Yaphe, J. and Ziebland, S. (2000) 'Database of patients' experiences (DIPEx): a multi-media approach to sharing experiences and information', *Lancet*, 355: 1540–3.

Hinton, T. (1994) 'Researching homelessness and access to health care', *Critical Public Health*, 5: 33–8.

Holden, P. (1991) 'Colonial sisters: nurses in Uganda', in P. Holden and J. Littlewood (eds), *Anthropology and nursing*. London: Routledge, pp. 67–83.

Homan, R. (1991) *The ethics of social research*. London: Longman.

Hughes, D. (1989) 'Paper and people: the work of the casualty reception clerk', *Sociology of Health and Illness*, 11: 382–408.

Inhorn, M. (1995) 'Medical anthropology and epidemiology: divergences or convergences?', *Social Science and Medicine*, 40: 285–90.

International Committee of Medical Journal Editors (1991) 'Uniform requirements for manuscripts submitted to biomedical journals', *British Medical Journal*, 302: 338–41.

Irigaray, L. (1985) *The sex which is not one*, trans. Catherine Porter with Carolyn Burke. Ithaca, NY: Cornell University Press.

James, M. (1994) 'Historical research methods', in K. McConway (ed.), *Studying health and disease*. Buckingham: Open University Press.

Jeffrey, R. (1979) 'Normal rubbish: deviant patients in casualty departments', *Sociology of Health and Illness*, 1: 90–107.

Jewkes, R., Abrahams, N. and Mvo, Z. (1998) 'Why do nurses abuse patients? Reflections from South African nursing obstetric services', *Social Science and Medicine*, 47: 1781–95.

Kaufert, P. (1988) 'Menopause as process or event: the creation of definitions in biomedicine', in M. Lock and D. Gordon (eds), *Biomedicine examined*. Dordrecht: Kluwer Academic Publishers, pp. 331–50.

Kendall, C., Foote, D. and Martorell, R. (1984) 'Ethnomedicine and oral rehydration therapy: a case study of ethnomedical investigation and program planning', *Social Science and Medicine*, 19: 253–60.

Khan, M.E. and Manderson, L. (1992) 'Focus groups in tropical diseases research', *Health Policy and Planning*, 7: 56–66.

Kitzinger, C. (1987) *The social construction of lesbianism*. London: Sage.

Kleinman, A. (1973) 'Toward a comparative study of medical systems: an integrated approach to the study of the relationship of medicine and culture', *Science, Medicine and Man*, 1: 55–65.

Krueger, R. and Casey, M.A. (2000) *Focus groups: a practical guide for applied research* (3rd ed.). Thousand Oaks, CA: Sage.

Lawler, J. (1991) *Behind the screens: nursing, somology and the problem of the body*. London: Churchill Livingstone.

Lawson, A. (1991) 'Whose side are we on now? Ethical issues in social research and medical practice', *Social Science and Medicine*, 32: 591–9.

Lenaghan, J. (1999) 'Involving the public in rationing decisions: the experience of citizens' juries', *Health Policy*, 49: 45–61.

Lévi-Strauss, C. (1966) *The savage mind*. Chicago: University of Chicago Press.

Lewando-Hundt, G. (2000) 'Multiple scripts and contested discourse in disseminating research findings', *Social Policy and Administration*, 34: 419–33.

Lewando-Hundt, G. (2001) ' "Good" reasons for "bad" records: the social, political and cultural context of vital registration', in M. MacLachlan (ed.), *Cultivating health: cultural perspectives on promoting health*. Chichester: John Wiley, pp. 37–53.

Lewando-Hundt, G., Abed, Y., Skeik, M., Beckerleg, S. and El Alem, A. (1999) 'Addressing birth in Gaza: using qualitative methods to improve vital registration', *Social Science and Medicine*, 48: 833–43.

Leydon, G. and Green, J. (2001) *The management of information in out-patient oncology consultations*. Final Report for ESRC, award number R000223142.

Leydon, G., Boulton, M., Moynihan, C., et al. (2000) 'Cancer patients' information needs and help seeking behaviour: an in depth interview study', *British Medical Journal*, 320: 909–13.

Lofland, J. (1971) *Analyzing social settings*. Belmont, CA: Wadsworth Publishing Company.

Lomax, H. and Casey, N. (1998) 'Recording social life: reflexivity and video methodology', *Sociological Research Online* 3(2) (http://www.socresonline.org.uk/socresonline/3/2/1.html).

Lupton, D. (1994) *Medicine as culture: illness, disease and the body in Western society*. London: Sage.

Madden, J.M., Quick, J.D., Ross-Degnan, D. and Kafle, K.K. (1997) 'Undercover careseekers: simulated clients in the study of health provider behaviour in developing countries', *Social Science and Medicine*, 45: 1465–82.

Mason, J. (1996) *Qualitative researching*. London: Sage.

Maynard, D. (1991) 'Interaction and asymmetry in clinical discourse', *American Journal of Sociology*, 97: 448–95.

Mays, N. and Pope, C. (1999) 'Quality in qualitative health research', in C. Pope and N. Mays (eds), *Qualitative research in health care* (2nd ed.). London: BMJ Books, pp. 89–101.

Mays, N., Roberts, E. and Popay, J. (2001) 'Synthesising research evidence', in N. Fulop, P. Allen, A. Clarke and N. Black (eds), *Studying the organisation and delivery of health services: research methods*. London: Routledge.

Meyer, J.E. (1993) 'New paradigm research in practice: the trials and tribulations of action research', *Journal of Advanced Nursing*, 18: 106–72.

Meyer, J.E. (1997) 'Action research in health care practice: nature, present concerns and future possibilities', *Nursing Times Research*, 2: 175–84.

Milburn, K., Fraser, E., Secker, J. and Pavis, S. (1995) 'Combining methods in health promotion research: some considerations about appropriate use', *Health Education Journal*, 54: 347–56.

Miles, M.B. and Huberman, A.M. (1994) *Qualitative data analysis: an expanded sourcebook* (2nd ed.). Thousand Oaks, CA: Sage.

Monaghan, L.F. (2003) 'Danger on the doors: bodily risk in a demonised occupation', *Health, Risk and Society*, 5: 11–32.

Morrow, V. and Richards, M. (1996) 'The ethics of social research with children: an overview', *Children and Society*, 10: 90–105.

Morse, J. (2002) 'A comment on comments', *Qualitative Health Research*, 12: 3–4.

Munodawafa, D., Gwede, C. and Mubayira, C. (1995) 'Using focus groups to develop HIV education among adolescent females in Zimbabwe', *Health Promotion International*, 10: 85–92.

Murphy, M.K., Black, N., Lamping, D.L., McKee, C.M., Sanderson, C.F.B., Askham, J., et al. (1998) 'Consensus development methods, and their use in clinical guideline development', *Health Technology Assessment*, 2(3): 1–88.

NCB (Nuffield Council on Bioethics) (2003) *The ethics of research related to healthcare in developing countries*. London: Nuffield Foundation.

Nettleton, S. (1992) *Power, pain and dentistry*. Buckingham: Open University Press.

Noblit, G.W. and Hare, R.D. (1988) *Meta-ethnography: synthesizing qualitative studies*. Newbury Park, CA: Sage.

Ntau, C.G. (2002) 'Medical careers of Botswana doctors' (Report from the Phil Strong Prize), *Medical Sociology News*, 28(3): 9–12.

Oakley, A. (1981) 'Interviewing women: a contradiction in terms?', in H. Roberts (ed.), *Doing feminist research*. London: Routledge, pp. 30–61.

Oakley, A. (1990) 'Who's afraid of randomised controlled trials?', in H. Roberts (ed.), *Women's health counts*. London: Routledge, pp. 167–94.

Ogden, J.A. and Porter, J.D.H. (2000) 'The politics of partnership in tropical public health: researching tuberculosis control in India', *Social Policy and Administration*, 34: 377–91.

Oinas, E. (1998) 'Medicalisation by whom? Accounts of menstruation conveyed by young women and medical experts in medical advisory columns', *Sociology of Health and Illness*, 20: 52–70.

O'Laughlin, B. (1998) 'Interpreting institutional discourses', in A. Thomas, J. Chataway and M. Wuyts (eds), *Finding out fast: investigative skills for policy and development*. London: Sage, pp. 107–26.

Opala, J. and Boillot, F. (1996) 'Leprosy among the Limba: illness and healing in the context of world view', *Social Science and Medicine*, 42: 3–19.

Paine, K., Hart, G., Jawo, M., et al. (2002) ' "Before we were sleeping, now we are awake": preliminary evaluation of the Stepping Stones sexual health programme in The Gambia', *African Journal of AIDS Research*, 1: 41–52.

Palmer, D. (2000) 'Identifying delusional discourse: issues of rationality, reality and power', *Sociology of Health and Illness*, 22: 661–78.

Patton, M.Q. (1990) *Qualitative evaluation and research methods* (2nd ed.). Newbury Park, CA: Sage.

Pelto, P.J. and Pelto, G.H. (1992) 'Developing applied medical anthropology in third world countries: problems and action', *Social Science and Medicine*, 35: 1389–95.

Peräkylä, A. and Silverman, D. (1991) 'Reinterpreting speech exchange systems: communication formats in AIDS counselling', *Sociology*, 25: 627–51.

Petticrew, M. (2001) 'Systematic reviews from astronomy to zoology: myths and misconceptions', *British Medical Journal*, 322: 89–101.

Plummer, K. (1983) *Documents of life: an introduction to the problems and literature of a humanistic method*. London: Unwin Hyman.

Pool, R. (1994) *Dialogue and the interpretation of illness: conversations in a Cameroon village*. Oxford: Berg.

Popay, J., Rogers, A. and Williams, G. (1998) 'Rationale and standards for the systematic review of qualitative literature in health services research', *Qualitative Health Research*, 8: 341–51.

Pope, C. (1991) 'Trouble in store: some thoughts on the management of waiting lists', *Sociology of Health and Illness*, 13: 193–212.

Potter, J. and Wetherell, M. (1987) *Discourse and social psychology: beyond attitudes and behaviour*. London: Sage.

Prior, L., Chun, P.L. and Huat, S.B. (2000) 'Beliefs and accounts of illness: views from two Cantonese-speaking communities in England', *Sociology of Health and Illness*, 22: 815–39.

Prior, P. (1995) 'Surviving psychiatric institutionalisation: a case study', *Sociology of Health and Illness*, 17: 651–67.

Rapley, T.J. (2001) 'The art(fulness) of open-ended interviewing: some considerations on analysing interviews', *Qualitative Research*, 1: 303–23.

Reason, P. (1998) 'Three approaches to participative inquiry', in N.K. Denzin and Y.S. Lincoln (eds), *Strategies of qualitative inquiry*. London: Sage, pp. 261–91.

Richards, L. (1999) *Using NVivo in qualitative research*. London: Sage.

Richardson, L. (2000) 'Evaluating ethnography', *Qualitative Inquiry*, 6: 253–5.

Richman, J. (2000) 'Coming out of intensive care crazy: dreams of affliction', *Qualitative Health Research*, 10: 84–102.

Rifkin, S. (1996) 'Rapid rural appraisal: its use and value for health planners and managers', *Public Administration*, 74: 509–26.

Ritchie, J. and Spencer, L. (1994) 'Qualitative data analysis for applied policy research', in A. Bryman and R.G. Burgess (eds), *Analyzing qualitative data*. London: Routledge, pp. 173–94.

Rogers, A. and Pilgrim, D. (1995) 'The risk of resistance: perspectives on the mass childhood immunisation programme', in J. Gabe (ed.), *Medicine, health and risk: sociological approaches*. Oxford: Blackwell, pp. 73–90.

Rosenhan, D.L. (1973) 'On being sane in insane places', *Science*, 179: 250–8.

Rowe, G. and Frewer, L.J. (2000) 'Public participation methods: a framework for evaluation', *Science, Technology and Human Value*, 25: 3–29.

Sackett, D.L., Rosenberg, W., Gray, J.A.M., Hayne, R.B. and Richardson, W.S. (1996) 'Evidence based medicine: what it is and what it isn't', *British Medical Journal*, 312: 71–2.

Sacks, H. (1989) 'Lecture four: an impromptu survey of the literature', *Human Studies*, 12: 253–9.

Scheper-Hughes, N. (2000) 'Ire in Ireland', *Ethnography*, 1: 117–40.

Schneider, H. and Palmer, N. (2002) 'Getting to the truth? Researching user views of primary health care', *Health Policy and Planning*, 17: 32–41.

Schwartzman, H. (1993) *Ethnography in organizations* (Qualitative Research Methods Series 27). London: Sage.

Scott, P. (1999) 'Black people's health: ethnic status and research issues', in S. Hood, B. Mayall and S. Oliver (eds), *Critical issues in social research*. Buckingham: Open University Press, pp. 80–93.

Scrimshaw, S.C.M. and Hurtado, E. (1988) 'Anthropological involvement in the Central American diarrheal disease control project', *Social Science and Medicine*, 27: 97–105.

Seale, C. (1999) *The quality of qualitative research*. London: Sage.

Shakespeare, T. (1999) ' "Losing the plot?": medical and activist discourses of contemporary genetics and disability', *Sociology of Health and Illness*, 21: 669–88.

Silverman, D. (1985) *Qualitative methodology and sociology*. Aldershot: Gower.

Silverman, D. (1993) *Interpreting qualitative data: methods for analysing talk, text and interaction*. London: Sage.

Silverman, D. (1998) 'The quality of qualitative health research: the open-ended interview and its alternatives', *Social Sciences in Health*, 4: 104–18.

Smith, D. (1988) *The everyday world as problematic: a feminist sociology*. Milton Keynes: Open University Press.

Smith, R. (1997) 'Authorship: time for a paradigm shift?', *British Medical Journal*, 314: 992.

Snowdon, C., Garcia, J. and Elbourne, D. (1997) 'Making sense of randomization: responses of parents of critically ill babies to random allocation of treatment in a clinical trial', *Social Science and Medicine*, 45: 1337–55.

Stern, G. and Kruckman, L. (1983) 'Multi-disciplinary perspectives on post-partum depression: an anthropological critique', *Social Science and Medicine*, 17: 1027–41.

Stimson, G. and Webb, B. (1975) *Going to see the doctor: the consultation process in general practice*. London: Routledge & Kegan Paul.

Stone, L. and Campbell, J.G. (1984) 'The use and misuse of surveys in international development: an experiment from Nepal', *Human Organization*, 43: 27–37.

Strauss, A. (1987) *Qualitative analysis for social scientists*. Cambridge: Cambridge University Press.

Strauss, A. and Corbin, J. (1990) *Basics of qualitative research: grounded theory procedures and techniques*. Newbury Park, CA: Sage.

Temple, B. (1997) 'Watch your tongue: issues in translation and cross cultural research', *Sociology*, 31: 389–408.

ten Have, P. (1999) *Doing conversation analysis: a practical guide*. London: Sage.

Thorogood, N. (1988) *Health and the management of daily life amongst women of Afro-Caribbean origin in Hackney*. University of London.

Thorogood, N. (1997) 'Questioning science', *British Dental Journal*, 183(5): 152–5.

Thoutenhoofd, E. (1998) 'Method in a photographic enquiry of being deaf', *Sociological Research Online*, 3(2) (http://www.socresonline.org.uk/socresonline/3/2/2.html).

Turner, V. (1967) *The forest of symbols: aspects of Ndembu ritual*. Ithaca, NY: Cornell University Press.

van der Geest, S. and Sarkodie, S. (1998) 'The fake patient: a research experiment in a Ghanaian hospital', *Social Science and Medicine*, 47: 1373–81.

VanderStaay, S.L. (2003) 'Believing Clayboy', *Qualitative Inquiry*, 9: 374–94.

Vissandjée, B., Abdool, S. and Dupéré, S. (2002) 'Focus groups in rural Gujarat, India: a modified approach', *Qualitative Health Research*, 12: 826–43.

Watts, S., Breiger, W. and Yacoob, M. (1989) 'Guinea worm: an in-depth study of what happens to mothers, families, and communities', *Social Science and Medicine*, 29: 1043–9.

Waxler-Morrison, N.E. (1988) 'Plural medicine in Sri Lanka: do Ayurvedic and Western medical practices differ?', *Social Science and Medicine*, 27: 531–44.

Webb, E.J., Campbell, D.T., Schwarz, R.D. and Sechrest, L. (1977) 'The use of archival sources in social research', in M. Bulmer (ed.), *Sociological research methods: an introduction*. London: Macmillan, pp. 113–30.

Wellings, K., Field, J., Johnson, A. and Wadsworth, J. (1994) *Sexual behaviour in Britain: the National Survey of Sexual Attitudes and Lifestyles*. Harmondsworth: Penguin.

Wenger, G.C. (1987) *The research relationship: practice and politics in social policy research*. London: Allen & Unwin.

West, P. (1990) 'The status and validity of accounts obtained at interview: a contrast between two studies of families with a disabled child', *Social Science and Medicine*, 30: 1229–39.

Whyte, W.F. (with K.K. Whyte) (1984) *Learning from the field: a guide from experience*. London: Sage.

Wilkinson, S. and Kitzinger, C. (2000) 'Thinking differently about thinking positive', *Social Science and Medicine*, 50: 797–811.

Winch, P. (1999) 'The role of anthropological methods in a community-based mosquito net intervention in Bagamoyo District, Tanzania', in R. Hahn (ed.), *Anthropology in public health: bridging differences in culture and society*. Oxford: Oxford University Press, pp. 44–62.

Wittig, M. (1992) *The straight mind and other essays*. Boston: Beacon.

WMA General Assembly (2000) *World Medical Association Declaration of Helsinki: ethical principles for medical research involving human subjects*.

Wolcott, H. (2002) 'Writing up qualitative work . . . better', *Qualitative Health Research*, 12: 91–104.

Wolff, B., Knodel, J. and Sittitrai, W. (1993) 'Focus groups and surveys as complementary research methods', in D. Morgan (ed.), *Successful focus groups: advancing the state of the art*. London: Sage, pp. 118–36.

Wright Mills, C. (1959) *The sociological imagination*. Oxford: Oxford University Press.

Yach, D. (1992) 'The use and value of qualitative methods in health research in developing countries', *Social Science and Medicine*, 35: 603–12.

Yin, R.K. (1994) *Case study research: design and methods* (2nd ed.). London: Sage.

Index